Sex clubs, non-monogamy, and game

The Red Quest

To Nash and to everyone who has shaped my thinking about
the game.

CONTENTS

Foreword

Sex clubs, non-monogamy, and game

There's little reason to read this book if you're not 1. already getting laid regularly and 2. confident in your ability to to meet and sleep with new women, or unusually intellectually curious. This book builds on a man's existing game; it isn't designed to teach the basics of game, since many other books already attempt to do just that. If you're a game newbie and don't have a girlfriend, start with Neil Strauss's classic *The Game*, or Geoffrey Miller and Tucker Max's *What Women Want*. Nick Krauser's books build on those two. There are many guides to picking up women, written by guys whose skills in that domain are superior to mine.

When you're able to get laid routinely, *then* read everything else here.

Sex clubs are not a shortcut to having real game. Sex clubs are an extension of existing game. If you don't have game and status already you will have a bad time if you try to bring your only, sole, everything-to-you girl to a sex club; if you invest your life savings in a single stock, you are one scandal away from going bankrupt, while a diversified portfolio or index fund ensures that you are financially robust. Girls are the same way, despite what the larger culture has told you about your need to find "the One" (she does not exist). If you bring your One Magic Girl to sex clubs, guys like me will try to pick her off. We might succeed. A guy who pins everything to one girl may go emotionally nuts the first time she has sex with another guy in front of him, or indicates that she wants sex with another guy (a later section of this book deals with jealousy). Before you bring a girl into that situation you need to know there's another one behind her, one you can access, if or when she bolts.

Normal guys can barely handle monogamy. For a guy to handle non-monogamy, he needs strong game skills and a strong frame.

The basic dynamic of sex parties is guys exchanging hot women with a minimal amount of logistical bother. That's it. People over-complicate and overthink this. You have a hot girl. I have a hot girl. Let's trade. The girl obviously has to like the other guy well enough (or want to fuck the girl).

Exchanging value for value is the game: I get more novelty than I'd have otherwise, while you get more novelty than you'd have otherwise. Win-win. Fail to bring the value and you will likely fail at the sex club. You get what you give. Guys who have a bad time with women in general will also have a bad time if they manage to convince their one and only partner to visit a sex club with them.

Single women sometimes come to sex clubs, and sometimes even attractive single women attend. Many guys will of course desire the single women for a threesome, and guys with sufficiently high status and good game are more likely to get them. Single women who are highly open to experience, are highly bisexual, or have very high sex drives are more likely to come on their own than average women. Most women, as players know, don't do shit unless there is a guy ready to lead them. Exceptions tend to be women with ultra-high libidos. Like, I've had a fairly long-term, off-and-on FWB who really, seriously wants to have sex twice a day, every day. You, the man reading this, may think, "Oh great mate, sign me up, I'd love to shag that much too." The vast majority of guys, especially guys over the age of 25, will eventually be knackered by a really persistent woman, and women who figure out their own sex drives realize they need multiple boyfriends or FWBs.

But the FWB I'm referencing is exceptional and unusual, and typical women at sex parties are brought by their primary partners. Typical guys want to swap with a girl who is at least on the level of the girl they've brought. It's about exchanging value, a phrase you'll read many times in this book.

The basics of game still apply to the non-monogamy world. Strong masculine identity and strong social skills lead to good outcomes. At parties and clubs, lots of guys try to get "something for nothing" by offering to swap with couples nowhere near their level. Usually they are declined. Occasionally, they do manage to swipe value from another guy, but this is rare; it's sort of like an average man getting laid by a much hotter woman because he's in the right place at the right time when she's horny. Can it happen? Sure. Is it repeatable and sustainable, like game? Nope. If a couple who are substantially below the level of my date and me wants to swap, I say no. If you bring a girl to a sex party, be ready to say "no."

Be ready to lead. Some chicks will lead themselves a little bit more as they get relaxed and into the sex zone, but most won't at the beginning. The fewer the people, the worse most chicks are at leading. So you, the man, will have to have the social deftness to make propositions and accept when they're rejected. And when they're accepted, which is scarier for some guys.

Women have the final say, and if a woman doesn't want to swap, it doesn't happen. "No means no" is important in the non-monogamy world. The club and party scene only works if there is no coercion and women can decline any sexual situation they do not like. More on this later.

Most cities have a "scene" of some kind. I don't know your city so I don't know what it entails. In your city, there will likely be a core nucleus of regulars, organizers, and people who make things happen. Show up enough and you will figure out who they are. Show up enough and you may become one of them by hosting your own events. If you're a high-value guy who regularly brings hot chicks, you'll be invited to events solo.

The worst clubs and parties are empty or filled with fatties or admit single men. I walk away from those events. When I use online app match systems, I emphasize my interests in lifting and fitness, and this acts as a fattie-repulsion system. Not perfectly, but well enough. The best response to a bad party is to walk out. Just because you have buy a ticket to a bad movie does not mean you must sit through it; just because you've bought a ticket to a sex club does not mean you are obligated to stay or have sex.

You know how girls who claim to have had bad experiences with men, usually have those experiences because they're totally drunk, or somewhere they shouldn't be, or doing something they shouldn't be? Same thing is true for couples who have bad experiences at sex clubs: the bad experiences rarely come out of nowhere and there is some kind of lead-up to the truly awful experience. Bad experiences arise when a couple at the club realizes that the club is admitting single men, or realizes there are too many people on drugs, or realizes that there are zero other couples or single women of interest. If any of those things are true, use your feet. A sex club or party may be dead on a given night, or may misrepresent itself. I have been invited to "parties" that end up consisting of one other couple, who I'm not interested in, and me and my date. When that happens, I take my date and depart. Before we go to a given event, I warn my date that the event might suck, and, if it does, we are going to leave. This sets reasonable expectations.

At the best events, there are many hot couples or, more rarely, unicorns—single, bisexual women. The hotter you are, the better you do. There is no such thing as a free lunch. Fantasize about a party full of gorgeous women aching for wild sex with you, but know that those don't exist in real life for normal guys. Because people are there for sex, guys can't hold out much in the way of resources and commitment to attract women. What Red Pill guys call "beta" or "nice guy" game works poorly. People are not there to find lifemates. They are there to have hot hot sex.

Lots of threeways have happened with women or couples I've met through the scene. If you're a reliable guy who brings hot girls in, you'll be in demand by other couples who want to swap. As you should know from reading Nancy Friday books, or some female-written erotica, lots of women fantasize about a threesome with two guys. Keep an eye out and you'll find other guys, possibly game-aware, who may become your go-to "threesome friend." You bring him in when you need a guy and vice-versa. It's all about the value. If you're providing value and he's providing value, you're golden.

At parties, calibrate your game to the scenario. Players, for example, are used to pushing through "maybe" girls in order to get them to "yes." This is typically a mistake at a party, where reputations are important and where a lot of chicks may be ambivalent. Ambivalence on a normal, one-on-one date can often be overcome. In a club or a couple-to-couple meet, assume anything other than "HELL YES" is a "no." Hold back more than push forward in this scene.

Most guys are poorly equipped, psychologically and physically, for the leadership role in a non-monogamous relationship, and most guys are poorly equipped to try out group sex. But the right guy, doing non-monogamy the right way, can be great. Like I said, he brings chicks, you bring chicks. He may have game, or he may just have a good social circle and persistence.

As for her, as for what your girl is thinking, most girls know that most men can't even articulate the girl's fantasies, let alone fulfill them. Being able to move her from fantasy to reality will blow her mind and simultaneously draw her into your world. "Wait!" you might be thinking, "How is it that a threesome with another guy will bring her closer to you?"

Simple: she's likely never been there before, and she knows that most guys will freak out if they hear her real fantasies. Girls usually lie to guys about their fantasies, because most guys cannot handle raunchy female fantasies. So any guy who can listen without judgment to her fantasies, or even propose the kind of sex she's dreamed about, must be special. It takes social finesse to make these things happen, and she'll know you have it, whereas other guys don't.

Most women legitimately fear that guys will shame them. Being a guy who doesn't slut shame and lets her explore her bedroom desires will set you apart. Most women never have their sexual fantasies fulfilled.

If you have a regular, uncommitted FWB you don't want for an LTR, try bringing her. Maybe you'll hate it. But it can be next-level game if you have the right stuff for it.

Most couples who come will be in committed relationships and they'll be a little bored with each other. If you're the guy who consistently brings in new hot women, you will be exceptional—a star. If you're in a casual, uncommitted relationship, you also know there's a decent chance she's f**king other people. Since she's probably doing it already, why not take her natural impulses and proclivities and make them work for you? Use what she's already doing to fuel your own sex life. It's like recycling conscientiously, but for sex.

Some women will say "no" to trying out a sex club, but many will be intrigued. I've been told many things. Like:

- You are too experimental.
- You are disgusting.
- I would never do something like that.
- I'm not that kind of girl.
- I want a guy who respects me.

The first one is my personal favorite. About a quarter of chicks have rejected me outright when I've proposed a sex club, (and I most often propose going after I've been sleeping with them for at least a couple weeks; for unusually adventurous girls I might talk about it on a first date. Depends on the girl). About a quarter have been excited and enthusiastic and don't need convincing. About half have been uncertain, but they will usually go if I encourage them and promise that we'll start slow.

Many sex parties and clubs will pretend to be egalitarian and "accept" (read: admit) people of all body types. Ignore the rhetoric. The reality is that sexual marketplace value operates at sex clubs, just like it does everywhere else. You cannot evade it. Using sex clubs to try to avoid having basic value and game will backfire and waste time. Guys who learn the game realize they need two things: value and a value delivery mechanism. Fail in either and the game won't work. At the clubs, you will very rarely see young girls who like the degradation of sex with gross, vile men. Most women assess men's sex appeal in all the usual ways.

I see almost no one writing about using open relationships and polyamory as a component of one's game ecosystem. To me, open relationships are, **used properly**, an extension of other kinds of game. Open relationships can lead to faster, hotter lays than opening girls on the street or online. Most guys aren't players. Most guys don't understand basic social dynamics. Most guys don't use or deploy open relationships properly, but most guys have no game and don't understand women at all, so they suffer.

A quick word on definitions: "Sex clubs" and "sex parties" are often used interchangeably. More strictly speaking, a "club" is usually an open invitation—take a club like Club Sapphire in Seattle or Whispers in Las Vegas. Almost anyone can attend, provided they are a single woman or a part of a couple.

Sex *parties* are usually more private. The most private are invite-only by the host. Less private ones may take over hotels or change venues regularly. They'll usually have a mailing list and usually operate only at specific times, like once a month. From the perspective of a game-aware guy, both venues can be appealing, depending on the night and on how connected he is in the community. Some parties will be held in private homes or condos, with the hosts doing some screening.

Sex parties can be open invitation, and many individuals or groups will put them on. But they're often closed to outsiders, and the only way to get in is through knowing people. In my experience, parties are usually better because the organizers have tight control over the guest list. The bigger the city, the better the scene, just like with normal game. Many guys have written me about how to get into sex clubs in rural areas or college towns. Answer: move.

This book is divided into two sections. The first is more like a textbook: it describes how non-monogamy works, why it works the way it does, and how skilled players can adopt aspects of non-monogamy into their game. The second section consists of stories around a key set of women who illustrate specific points or were key in my own development. There are other stories I could tell, but I wasn't writing about most of these experiences contemporaneously. Because of that, many of the finer details have washed away. I have had many other cares in my life, and it was not until recently that I began to explain what I've learned.

The world is changing. I don't think I saw any articles or books about non-monogamy until about five years ago— around 2014 or 2015. Today, they appear routinely. When I started, it was rare to find girls or couples age 20 - 25 in the scene. Today, it's far more common. Many people know that the person they're dating early in their lives will not be the person they marry, so why not experiment? As these ideas diffuse through society, we're likely to see this world expand.

In addition to the book you're about to read, you may also find my novel, *The Good Girl*, worth reading: instead of the textbook approach pursued here, it's a story. Humans learn via stories more than they do via direct instruction, so I'd recommend you read it too.

This book is also a record of sex adventures. Along the way, I had many other cares and tasks, and those aren't recorded here, and what is recorded is a particular set of activities and interests. Because I don't mention other hobbies or interests, doesn't mean they don't exist. Some women and couples I initially met through sex, and eventually the sex fell away, while the friendship remained. Some women and couples were initially friends, and the sex came months or years or breakups later. I'm not (solely) a sex machine. Sometimes, the sex happened very fast, within minutes or hours of meeting. Sometimes it came slowly, after many hours together at clubs or parties or movies or dinners. Given the subject matter of this book, it will probably not be a surprise that, all else equal, I preferred sex with attractive women happen sooner rather than later, but life often doesn't work out the way I'd most prefer. Most women want to be seen as people, not purely as sex objects, and seeing a woman as a person will often let her want to be seen and taken in a highly sexual way. Letting a woman know you see her as a person often takes time.

I'm also not explicitly advocating for consensual non-monogamy, threesomes, or group sex. I am, however, trying to help men understand the sexual marketplace; help men understand female psychology; help men perceive the possibilities that are out there; help men leverage "sex positive" culture; and help men improve their efficiency. Consensual non-monogamy has enriched my life. It has trade-offs, but it also has rewards, and I've seen few men discuss how the scene works, what to expect, how to get in it, and what principles drive it. Other men have effectively covered many aspects of game. I've decided to cover this one.

CHAPTER ONE

How the non-monogamy game works

Consensual non-monogamy is harder to pitch to the average chick than one-on-one dating, but in my opinion it's more honest—especially for players, many of whom don't want or won't accept a monogamous girlfriend. Beyond honesty, non-monogamy may be more efficient, too, although about a quarter of girls dump me or flat out refuse when I mention it. About a quarter are gung-ho. Half are ambivalent and can be amenable to non-monogamy, if it's pitched correctly. I don't think it's wise to bring up non-monogamy until you've been sleeping together for a while and she's firmly converted into your frame. Players know the tipping point when a chick flips from evaluating the man for sex to knowing the man is evaluating her for a relationship. For most chicks, it's valuable to get past that point before dropping the sex-club bomb.

Three very good sex sessions is a rule of thumb for strong conversion, but every guy must learn for himself how to feel out conversion. Some girls are also fundamentally non-monogamous in a masculine way, and they will never be deeply converted into a man's frame... some guys don't want to recognize this but it's true.

Neil Strauss's *The Game* sequel, *The Truth* (a great book, though you may disagree with the end), has him exploring non-monogamy:

> *I look up and see a yoga stud from Kamala's pod.*
> *"Have you rounded up any more girls?" the orbiter asks him.*
>
> *Kamala Devi and Shamal Helena said polyamory was about loving relationships, not casual sex. But these guys seem more like next-level pickup artists, coming to these conferences with the intention of sucking any available women into their powerful reality.*

"These guys seem more like next-level pickup artists:" let that sink in.

Why haven't pick-up artists figured this out? It more efficient to sleep with girls this way.

People who have too much time to contemplate their open relationships get very excited about the terms they use and the connotations from those terms. I don't get hung up on the particular terms "poly" or "open" because I don't care that much. If the label "poly" lets me keep a girl on rotation for a longer period of time as a friend-with-benefits or lover, because she knows my love is too great for only a single person… just like hers… that's fine with me (and that has happened to me). Good sex without obligation on my part? Okay, yeah, sure, whatever it takes, yeah, I'm poly. Pass the joint, will you?

Other people, usually of a more ideological type, want to break down the differences among open relationships, and there are three main avenues involved in non-monogamous relationships:

* * *

- **Polyamory**: Polyamorous people have long-term, deep, attached romantic relationships with more than one person. Think of a trio of people in a single relationship with set boundaries.
- **Swingers**: Swingers have sex with other people, typically couple-to-couple, but don't form deep romantic relationships with other people. They tend to have "friends with benefits." No one expects financial cross-subsidies, or no moreso than a given couple would with their friends.
- **Open Relationships**: People who are simply "open" are allowed to go have sex with other people, in pairs or individually.

I never use the word "swinger" because it's been polluted by '60s and '70s associations. If I hear "swinger" from others, I ignore it. I usually prefer not to discuss the idea of open relationships overtly. Instead, I like to invite a girl to a "sex party." That phrase sounds better. "Sex club" also sounds a little too '70s for most girls, and "the club" has a set of associations I also don't necessarily want to activate. If I invite a girl to a sex party before she springs "the talk," she may break up with me before the talk. Or, if we do have the talk, she already has context for an open relationship, which is useful for me. I also like the terms "sex-positive" and "consensual non-monogamy," since they haven't been polluted by '70s associations.

I've rarely seen attractive polyamorous people who wish to generally advertise that they are polyamorous. But I have seen lots of attractive open relationship people, particularly among those who identify as "swingers." Remember, though, that there is no escape from frame or SMV. If the former is strong and the latter is high it can be next-level game.

* * *

Where you live matters

Like game itself, the quality and quantity of non-monogamous relationships will vary based on location. The bigger the city, the better the scene. New York appears to have the best scene in the United States. I've heard from guys in cities like St. Louis, Boise, and Baltimore that there are no good sex clubs nearby and that the online dating world is a wasteland. A few of those guys imply I'm lying about my own good experiences. The best advice for many guys who want to be in the game is, "Move." Guys living in distant suburbs or small cities are going to have a harder time in the game itself and a far harder time convincingly doing non-monogamy, because there are too few options. The smaller the city, the greater the social surveillance. In a big city like New York, or even a medium-sized city like Portland, enough people flow in and out to ameliorate the surveillance issue while also ensuring there are always new chicks to date. Girls in small towns and small cities have to protect their reputations, since everybody knows everybody. In big cities, that's far less true, so it's much more possible to have hot, anonymous sex with attractive strangers—without social repercussions.

Couples interested in non-monogamy need to be able to find other couples on their level. We all have a level of some kind; we're all familiar with this from normal dating. A girl who walks into a club and sees no one she considers closer to her level may be permanently turned off by the scene.

I've also taken smart girls on dates with couples who are okay to look at but who are stupid. Smart girls won't compromise that much and often demand guys and couples who are at her intellectual level. For a hot girl, however, I'm willing to compromise on intellect for short-term flings—just like most guys.

A book called *Date-onomics* by blue-pill writer Jon Birger

describes how even subtle changes in sex ratios between men and women can create very different dating outcomes. Men in San Francisco and Seattle are surrounded by guys who can afford the real estate and move to be in the tech industry. Women are scarce, so monogamy is more common and women have more market power. New York City and Boston are the opposite: women move there to work in media, fashion, etc., so there are far more women than men. A man interested in non-monogamy should choose NYC if he can, or the next-biggest cities if he can't, such as Chicago or Los Angeles. If he needs to stay in particular state or region, he should move to the largest city in the state or region. If he's in Tennessee or any of the surrounding states, he should try for Nashville. Same thing with Atlanta and Georgia.

Not for everyone

I have never said (and will never say) that "non-monogamy is for everyone" or "group sex is great for everyone." It's not and it's not. But, given how most players like sexual novelty and variety, and given that most women in uncommitted relationships are going to be f**king around anyway, a guy should consider some of these strategies as a way of achieving better output for less work while also retaining the girl better. "Retention" is a surprising issue to many players, but a lot of girls want sexual novelty too, just like guys do. A lot of girls feel the tension between their desires to have sex with multiple guys and their desires to have a primary relationship. Non-monogamy is intensely desirable to some girls, too.

Non-monogamy and sex parties are dangerous to a primary relationship, as they offer a girl up to potential poachers. But non-monogamy and sex parties also offer an incredible test of a girl: is she truly loyal to you, or is she loyal out of convenience? If she goes off with some guy who d**ks her well, then she was likely never that loyal in the first place. For a player, the big advantage of the scene is variety. And the degree to which a guy can make fast friends should not be underestimated. Friendship emerges from shared interests and perspective. Many friendships are born out of this scene. I don't want to overemphasize this aspect, as there is plenty of competition involved, as you will see.

To me, non-monogamy is a faster, more honest way of achieving hot sex. Some guys do daygame. Others, nightgame (which has never been good for me). Others, online (where competition is ridiculous and fierce).

It's also surprising to me that more players haven't figured non-monogamy out. Maybe I'm lazier than some players and like having some of the filtering work done for me, in advance. Girls in sex clubs obviously self-select for being libidinous and sex-positive. But I think guys also make a fundamental conceptual mistake: in my view, there are only two kinds of relationships: one that lead to a man and woman having children together, and all other kinds. Most people treat "all other kinds" too much like relationships in which "a man and woman have children together." Mine is not a common view, however. If you want to have children with a particular woman, then do not introduce her to non-monogamy. Most men do not want to have children with most women, so the child issue is irrelevant.

Some players are driven by the ego-based thrill of accomplishment they get from hot chicks, which is also fine, and that ego-thrill makes them chase one-night stands. I'm thrilled by sex itself with pretty girls. There is probably some ego involved for me, but I don't think it's my primary drive. I'm not trying to make a value judgment about ego, but guys who make it past the opening stages of the game often ask, "What's driving me?", because the answer will affect what he's doing and how he's doing it. Guys like me, who really love the physical act itself without caring as much about the buildup to it, may like the sex-positive, non-monogamy scene better than guys who love the feeling of accomplishment that comes from executing a difficult task (like f**king a hot, bitchy girl who seems indifferent early in the seduction).

What you'll hear

Many people in non-monogamy erroneously present it as being about the harmonious coming together of disparate people in a jealousy-free environment that transcends the boundaries and possessiveness of traditional relationships. They say it's about achieving a higher level of consciousness. It's about realizing that sex is beautiful and that we can create more beautiful sex in the world through overcoming our limitations. They say jealousy is a social construct, as is monogamy.

In reality, most people experience jealousy; most people seek value and will tap value without paying for it if they can (and if they think they can get away with it). In reality, most attractive women who have sex with a large number of strange men are getting paid. The way you'll hear non-monogamy presented is not totally inaccurate, because there are people who practice non-possessiveness, who are willing to give much more than they receive, and who subsidize hot chicks.

There are counterintuitive ideas involved in this world, like that women will bond to a man because of his ability to fulfill her fantasies, or that women experience jealousy and deep emotional connection with a man while she is being promiscuous and so is he. But most people in the non-monogamy scene are still sensitive to reciprocity, to the fear of being alone, to the need for companionship, and to the values of the sexual marketplace. Many domains in human social life have a surface set of explanations that people espouse, and beneath the surface a real set of explanations that drive behavior. I'm working to illuminate the latter, while still occasionally gesturing to the former.

One guy wrote to me, "Before I read your book, I thought sex clubs to be drunken, bacchanalian parties filled with drugs. Your descriptions make them seem much more like friendly social gatherings where people have expert manners. That actually makes a lot more sense because there needs to be 'hidden rules' in place for this sort of ecosystem to be sustainable." Exactly. Almost no large and public sex clubs allow drunks or people who use drugs to excess, or to the point that they violate other people's space and desires. Sex clubs only work if women feel safe and men know their dates won't be molested. Take away the safety and the club will swiftly die, for good reason. People who violate the rules will quickly be ostracized (again, for good reason). No one wants to have their value stolen and failure to enforce rules leads to the high value of hot women being stolen.

Think of rock climbing. Rock climbing is inherently dangerous. The people who do it successfully (and don't die) are often very conservative about equipment, weather, and training. They make absolutely sure their safety gear is top notch and in good working order. If they see signs the weather is turning, they turn back, even if the summit is close. They train hard to consecutively reach more difficult mountains, glaciers, or rock faces, and no one smart starts with Everest, K2, or even Denali. Something similar can be said for sex parties: the people who do it successfully often plan their evenings and dates. They decide what their limits and rules are for a given night. If they want to change the rules for their next date or club, they can. They check in with their partners. If something seems off about new partners, they disengage. And the people who do sex clubs successfully look for others who share the same ethic. Drink and drugs that impair one's ability to function properly and to respect others are not going to work with these needs. Manners and etiquette, however, help people structure interactions. Being too mannered is stultifying, but not being mannered enough is rude or confusing. People who are successful in a given situation learn to operate between those poles.

Bringing a chick to the party for the first time

There's no single way I introduce chicks to group sex and open relationships, because every chick is a little different and needs different calibration. I rarely introduce the idea of sex parties to a girl until we've had sex enough times that we're regulars with each other. The process from cold open to lay is well-described elsewhere, and my own cold approach skills are mediocre; I also like medium-term relationships with chicks and find that the best parts of many relationships happen from about two weeks in until the end of the second year: the sex is still very hot, the girl is still very novel (and the guy is novel to her), and most people remain on good behavior. It's often difficult to retain girls after the first two or three months, though, because most girls want, or think they want, to be "boyfriend and girlfriend" by that point, which can dampen a guy's ability to be in the game and achieve sexual novelty. To me, bringing the girl into the group-sex scene is a way of maintaining her in my orbit while also sleeping with new chicks. The girl can also be leveraged for sex with new girls.

The first girl who brought me into the scene, "Libido Girl," is unusual and I've not met many chicks like her (her story is in the second section of this book). Since she got me into the sex-positive, non-monogamous community, I've brought a bunch of chicks to clubs, to parties, and on dates with other couples, and there's a finesse to introducing first-timers. A chick who is super sex-positive will be different than a chick who is sex-negative or comes from a highly religious background.

My personal vibe is also open to experience and non-judgmental, and that will make the girl more honest about what she's into and what she's done. I'm confident many chicks still lie to me, or omit key details and desires—which is fine, but they see what I do in bed and how I talk to them. In bed I use collars, restraints, blindfolds, floggers, and paddles. I like making sex tapes. I put buttplugs into girls and then watch their whole bodies convulse with feeling when we have sex. To me all that stuff is normal, to the point now that I forget most chicks aren't used to a full-body, all out experience. I tend to bring stuff out a little too quickly, leading to the, "Do you do this with every girl?" question.

(Typical response: "I look at sex as the ultimate experience and am with you, here, right now, and we're learning about each other. I'm figuring out what you like and respond to. We're in this together, and we're exploring." This basic suite of ideas overcomes that question, which can be a shit test but is really I think the chick being worried about me being a player and being worried about her just being another number. Which she often is, but we'll leave that to the side.)

When I'm prepping a new chick, I'll ask her about threesomes. What was her first threesome like? That phrasing is crucial: if a guy asks **if** she's had a threesome, she's less likely to admit it than if he asks how her first threesome was. Some chicks will say they haven't had one. If they have had threesomes, I'll ask, "How'd it go?" What were her partners like? If they haven't had one, I'll ask if they've fantasized about them. Girls typically won't lead and won't act on their fantasies unless there is a guy or a rare girl who will lead to make the fantasies happen.

Usually the girl will reciprocate and ask about my experiences, and I'll tell her about my first threesome and one or two other key experiences. I emphasize the idea that a girl in a threesome typically has an amazing experience because all the attention is on her. Chicks love attention. Two people kissing her, two people on her neck, one one her neck another going down on her, etc. In a sexually charged environment, like being nude in bed with the chick, this is often highly arousing to her.

Eventually, often weeks or sometimes a month or longer after the threesome talk and fantasy probes, I'll drop the bomb and say, "I know this sex club, and we should go." "Some people are having a sex party, and I want you to come with me." Chicks rarely say yes immediately. They'll usually have a barrage of questions about what it's like, how I got into it, what I know about it, will I have sex with another chick there. But chicks, at least chicks I'm with and the chicks I have seeded properly, rarely reject the idea outright, either. Remember that it's important for the chick to be sexually bonded before a guy brings this idea up. Her reciprocity goes up after she's invested in you. Sometimes I'll make the inquiry overly soon... that isn't optimal, but if a guy senses a girl is deeply into him quickly, it can be done. If I'm not that into the girl, I may propose the sex club much sooner, because if she's super enthusiastic my view of her might rise. Even if it turns out to not be for her, I get reputational credit for bringing a new girl to the sex club.

When I introduce the sex-club idea to a chick, I emphasize fantasy: it's about us living out her fantasies and exploring what she really likes. Most chicks, I think, have a robust fantasy life they're too scared to seek out and make real.

Evolution has bequeathed most chicks with a certain surface conservatism. Most chicks who are passive still get to reproduce… some guy will come along and seduce her or make her his, and her genes will get into the next generation.

There is genetic evidence for this, because geneticists have found that we're descended from about eighty percent of the women who have ever reached reproductive age and about forty percent of the men. The average guy died without issue. The average chick had some babies. Chicks subconsciously know that they don't have to try and should probably not try most things on their own. Better to let the man go first into the new environment, the dark cave, etc. This is why chicks start fewer companies and far fewer chicks become important artists or scientists. Nothing drives them out to the bleeding edge. Guys know, subconsciously, that if we don't strive, our entire lineage dies out. Better to take the risk and reap the rewards than play it safe. To quote philosopher and hero Camille Paglia, "If civilization had been left in female hands we would still be living in grass huts." Many guys don't understand how cosseted the average woman's world is and how little that matters to the average woman, because she's content following a man's lead.

Chicks look to guys for guidance about what to do and how to behave. This is also why guys who don't learn how to lead will **never** get their sex lives to where their sex lives should be. A lot of game is just learning to tolerate rejection, have social sense, and then lead a chick through the steps and into your bed. Chicks rarely take affirmative, direct actions to make their sex lives better. Instead, they wait for a guy to come along and make their lives happen. Chicks also sometimes look to each other for leadership, which is why a group of girls is so funny to watch: no one will make a decision because every chick wants someone else to make the decision.

As a younger guy, I didn't understand why chicks won't be proactive. Now I get it and have adjusted my behavior accordingly.

Most chicks are not very sexually experimental, **on the surface**. Many exceptions exist, but game should target the median hot chick, and then game should be calibrated to the individual girl's temperament. A deft guy can often bring chicks into his reality and do the things with her that she'll deny to her friends and sometimes even herself. ("It's not me who's in charge, he's just making me do this.") Giving a chick plausible deniability is a good way to get her into bed. That's why no one says, "Do you want to come back to my place for sex?" It's always, "I have a bottle of wine." "Let's go watch a movie." "Let's play guitar." When the chick says, "Okay, but I'm not having sex with you," the guy says, "Who said anything about sex? It's interesting that that's on your mind." Etc., etc. Standard game things.

The average chick has a stronger need for security, safety, and social approval than the average guy. Chicks worry deeply about what their friends and family will think of them, and what future men will think of them, and those worries may prevent the girl from exploring her sexual urges. As a man, your job is to reassure her that she is still "good," that the event will be fun, and that her friends and family don't need to know about what she's doing. Most women would rather remain socially acceptable than have peak experiences. Your job is to navigate those waters and help the woman understand that it's normal and fun to be sexually explorative. You will keep her secure and safe. Her position with you is safe and secure and will be enhanced by having these experiences. Reinforcing such ideas may take time.

The first chick I took to a club, after Libido Girl introduced me, was someone I'd met previously at a business / networking event. I'd seen her for a while before Libido Girl, then she'd broken it off (I didn't know how to handle non-monogamy then and was just getting properly disentangled from a long-term partner) and she'd boomeranged back as Libido Girl and I were ending our affair. I took this girl to a party being held by friends, where she loved having another girl go down on her, then to a club, and that's when this whole thing began to click for me: I figured out or consciously realized that parties are mostly about guys who want to trade chicks and thus get lots of casual sex on "easy mode." I also learned that Libido Girl wasn't singular and that the practices I was developing were repeatable.

The process was not quite that easy because to make sex clubs work, the guy has to be attractive, socially skilled, and bring the hot chick in the first place. But if he has those elements in place... the sex part naturally flows. I've been to good parties where my girl and I have hit it off with another couple, and within fifteen minutes I'm deep in the other girl. With a first-time girl, however, it's useful to frame the sex club by saying you're going to check it out together, and you're not going to have sex with anyone else. This reduces the pressure. Smart couples do this in general; in couples that blow up, one person often wants to hit the accelerator while the other wants to hit the brake. Couples who last go at the pace of the slower person.

The most interesting girl I brought is probably the one I call "SA Girl:" she was a high 8 or maybe low 9 but didn't act, or dress, like it, and I think she was young enough to not fully appreciate her sexual market value (SMV). She was also introverted and didn't behave in the hot young bitchy girl way, so we were uncommonly compatible. A guy who brings a stunning chick to a sex club will forever be the guy who can get hot chicks, thus opening many interesting experiences and doors.

* * *

How entering the sex party feels, and how most sex parties are structured, is covered in the chapter "Socializing and culture at sex clubs."

Some girls will initially say "no," hard, to sex clubs. You can persist a bit, by giving her dates, times, projecting an active fantasy with her there, etc., but if she remains a hard no it's time to move on to other girls. Most modern chicks will be open to the new experience, as long as it's with a guy they already like and trust.

Today, the worst thing a guy can be is boring. If you propose taking her to the sex club, you are unlikely to be seen as boring. If you've been on some dates with a girl but can feel her interest slipping, a sex-club bomb might make her swing back around. Talk to enough chicks and you'll hear them say how boring and straightforward most guys are. Most girls are bored and boring, so they respond well to stimulating novelty from a guy they know well enough to trust. Game teaches you to be that guy. I am helping you take that guy to the next level.

Leadership: women want to follow your lead

Years ago I dated this average-but-pretty woman, and I slowly introduced her to sex-positive culture and sex parties. When we first started dating she presented a fairly average relationship and sex history, but she was intrigued by exhibitionism and us fucking together with other people around us and, over the course of a month or two, I got her to go to a sex party with me. She became comfortable with the scene and people. After four or five parties, she was ready to swap partners; this pattern became normal for me, but at the time it was novel and I was not sure how well it would work or how many chicks would be willing to seek sexual adventure. That was hard for her at first, and about half of women I've gotten to do this find it very hard, while about half are pretty curious to try contrary to some of the man-o-sphere descriptions, which depict women as wanton harlots, most women are not wanton harlots, though they can be in the right circumstance. This woman did do it and over time she became more sex-positive. In her rhetoric and actions she began to favor group sex and consensual non-monogamy.

Eventually things soured because I wouldn't move in with her and refused to make a long-term commitment… a long time ago I decided that cohabitation is not for me, and refusing the "next steps" has probably been the end of my last 10 – 15 short- to medium-term relationships (eventually I recanted on that, but only after many years of refusing to move a relationship forward). Most women have their own dating timeline and it moves from meeting to kissing to casual sex to deep sex to moving in, marrying, and children. Then she gets bored, divorces the guy, takes half his money. Or he gets bored, finally bangs someone he meets at work, gets found out, divorces anyway. Few of us can handle getting everything we've ever wanted.

My timeline, however, stops at deep sex and most women will break up with me when I tell them after a couple months that there is no "next" step to the relationship. It is possible to lie and let women dangle for long periods of time, but I think it's mean, deceptive, and hurts both the woman and the guy telling the lie. Women also have tight reproductive timelines and for women over the age of 30 it's cruel to let them invest years of their reproductive prime in a relationship that isn't going anywhere.

Plus, if you let a woman age 30+ invest years of her reproductive prime in you, don't be surprised if she takes matters into her own hands and "forgets" to take her birth control. Or she gets her IUD out and doesn't have it replaced.

You may argue it's unethical for a woman to "accidentally" get pregnant from a guy she's casually seeing. I agree. It's also unethical and cruel to let a woman invest years of her reproductive prime at age 30+ in a relationship that won't lead to kids. Yes, she should "know better," but so should you. Have fun with her for a couple months, then be straightforward about being a player and not wanting kids (or kids with her).

Point of the story is, I did like this woman and I did like the way she had sex. She was willing to be led into the sex party part of my social life, and, because I didn't push her too hard, over time she came to really love it.

Like most women who breakup for timeline issues, we kept hooking up for a while. In these situations it's common for the woman to find another guy, date him, break up with him, and come back for more sex. I kept taking her to sex clubs, although she would have moral hangovers after.

I don't think any of her friends totally knew what we were up to, although some could read between the lines when they'd ask what we were doing and I'd say things like, "Going to a party," and when they'd ask if they could come, I'd explain that I'm not sure it was for them and that I wasn't the host. If you do this kinda shit with a smile you can get away with it. Some of them would drunkenly confide their own dark sex desires to me, because they knew I'd keep those desires secret.

Recently, this guy I distantly work with acquired a new girlfriend. One night I finally meet her and it's the same one from my story! Just older. Meeting was awkward for her and for him, because the girl and I obviously knew each other. I just did my usual thing in this circumstance and was like, "Oh hey, I remember you from Joe's party." Women want to fall into your frame and she fell right into mine again, saving face and making sure it's less awkward than it would be otherwise for the guy dating her.

Part of the reason this encounter went more smoothly than it could have is because she knows I don't want to shame her in front of her new man. I don't want to out her. She knows that my sex positivity is real. She acquiesced to taping sex acts that could be viewed as degrading because she knew, correctly, that I would never use those tapes against her.

Some snippets of those tapes are still on the Internet but she is not identifiable. If you are part of the secret society and really keep the "secret" part of the secret society, good things will happen to you. The "secret society" is a concept originated by a guy from Real Social Dynamics (RSD)—Tyler, I think. He says:

> *A secret society exists. Around 52% of people on this earth are a part of it. In the 52%, 50% are women, 2% are men.*
>
> *Of the 2% of male members, half are gay, the other half are players. What I'm talking about is the sex secret society - and you are either IN or OUT .*
>
> *SOME RULES OF THE SECRET SOCIETY:*
>
> *1) Don't talk about the secret society.*
>
> *2) The priority of the secret society is to have perpetually good emotions in all members.*
>
> *3) Create shrouds around the secret society, like "all men are dogs". Hide the truth that women are far more likely to cheat than men.*
>
> *4) If you are part of the secret society, you will never be denied anything at any point.*
>
> *5) If you are not part of the secret society, you will scrap and beg for everything you get.*
>
> *6) Communication in the secret society is less often verbal, and more often spoken through body language subcommunications, and verbal subcommunications that*

would only make sense to members. Any other way, and the 48% of men would pick up on it, and it would no longer be a secret.

7) At the first sign that someone who is not part of the secret society is possibly trying to pretend that he is, berate him with both love-rhetoric, and accusations of chauvinism and nit-witted-ness.

Men outside the secret society don't understand the nature of women. They don't understand how carnal women can, and prefer, to be. Secret society members also understand that reputations need to be maintained, and, for that reason, female members of the secret society prefer not to have their membership outed or discussed. Women at sex parties don't want their families, or their future provider guys, to know they've attended.

Women will make sex tapes with dominant men, but they will often ask that those sex tapes be deleted as part of the breakup process, as she purges her past, "bad" self, and prepares for her "good" future self, who has always been monogamous and always will be. Women know they may need to later marry a clueless guy who is bad in bed but financially adequate. A woman does not want that beta guy to see tangible evidence of her being passionate and orgasmic with another man, and she does not want her financial provider to see her engaged in acts she might not engage in with him. She may fake orgasm with him. She doesn't want him to suspect that his children might not be his after all.

But women do want the pleasure of sex with a dominant, sexy guy who might not commit. The secret society admits those women and they know their own desires and drives, even as they deny those desires and drives to others. The key is to give women plausible deniability. I don't tell a woman's friends she's been going to sex parties. I let her do that on her own. She often will, usually after a couple drinks, and only with her girlfriends. I don't know how much this woman told to her friends, but I do know she went from thinking that sex parties were a bizarre aberration to participating in them with me. More women are up for this than the average guy thinks. What's possible is partly defined by our view of ourselves, and what we think is possible. Men's understanding of women is largely dependent on who they're able to attract and retain, and how effectively they're able to lead. Most men present a "monogamous" mindset and culture, and try to restrict women's sexuality, and, as a consequence, most women present that way, even if they're willing to do other things and behave other ways. My view of reality is different and many women are willing to enter my world, if I present it properly and read it properly.

I'm 95% sure she's not going to tell the guy she's dating that she's fucked me and fucked a bunch of other guys and gals with me. I'm pretty sure my colleague has a normal frame and worldview about women that does not include understanding that women love sex and will do almost anything for a guy they really want to keep. He likely can't imagine this woman partner-swapping and fucking a guy whose name she doesn't even know while I do the same to a girl. I feel kinda bad for the guy, but it's not my job to wake him up; that's his job. He's a fine guy overall but he presents to women as weak and normal so I'm sure women treat him that way.

He should know or suspect her history, but his mind doesn't want to go there. People can tell which guys are players and which guys are losers who can't get dates, and while I've mostly stopped bringing dates to most company or industry functions, people know. I try to minimize that reputation because it doesn't help me for the most part, but it is not possible to fully hide who you are.

I want to be a hedonistic slut and, over time, demand that women do the same. My colleague probably wants women to present as demure, and so his dates present that way. Social "truths" depend on context. Most people do not actually stand for anything, so they follow the lead of the strongest person they see. A woman will follow a man's lead all kinds of places if the man knows what he wants and can show her that it is a good thing to want and do. Most men want nothing true, or cannot adequately pursue what they think they want, and their outcomes are consistent with that.

To quote another writer, "Your woman is pretty much malleable to whatever values or life you to intend to live, if your frame is strong enough." If you have that strong frame a lot becomes possible. Most women hide their deep sexual desires for fear of being judged by other women and by men. The number who will speak about how they feel or act out their fantasies is small because most women are constrained by the box other women and men put around them. I try to open that box.

Show her what type of man you are so she knows what kind of woman to be.

Someone asked me whether most guys in non-monogamous relationships are secretly or overtly bisexual. I don't think so, and guys who are bi or want to experiment with men can go to any gay bar any night of the week to do so. They don't need to go to a straight sex club, which is a venue where women can explore and explore with other women in a positive-reinforcement environment. Gay guys do what straight guys wish they could and have sex all the time. So there's really no need for them to go through the whole party and club process that straight group sex entails. A guy who wants to experiment with other men doesn't need all the effort. He can put up a Grindr profile that says,

"Predominantly straight bi guy looking to experiment." Within an hour he'll be able to experiment as much as he wants. For gay guys, "a sex party" is also just known as "Friday night at Steve's place."

Many girls are bi. Maybe more say they are bi than are actually bi. It could be that girls say they're bi in order to reduce female-female competition.

Frame and non-monogamy

As guys who get deeply into the game know, the initial parts of game are about attraction and dominance, but most chicks tell themselves that they can eventually tame the bad boy and turn him into a long-term provider-guy—that is basically the plot of all romance novels and romance novels are porn for women. Even among players who imply or explicitly say to women that they're only in it for the casual sex, lots of women will fantasize about locking those guys down long-term, or the women will attempt it, as long as the guy has an okay job.

In addition, most normal women eventually want children and most normal women also want to be financially subsidized by a guy. If the guy is also hot and good in bed, that's a plus, but for a long-term provider it may not be necessary. This conflict between short-term hots and long-term provision is fundamental and explained by evolutionary biology.

Even among women who are being picked up on the street, an element of "will this guy be my long-term provider?" often arises at some point. Initially it may be and probably will be all about the seduction and the hot sex, and most guys underperform in being hot, dominant, and playful because society teaches them to do the opposite.

But over time that biological need to find a guy for kids,

and a guy who will subsidize her and her kids, becomes acute. That's part of the reason long-term, undefined, FWBs-type relationships are so uncommon. Few chicks will allow them, at least past the age of 25. Even if they do, they will drop the FWB when they find a hot-enough provider guy.

(If you're dating a chick under the age of 25 in a contemporary Western country, you can ignore the last two paragraphs, because chicks that age are all about the feelz and the hot sex.)

This is useful background because, at sex parties, *the provider part of the equation goes away almost entirely*, at least for a night of passion. The chick probably already has a primary partner who she evaluates in part for his material characteristics. The new guy needs to primarily be a hot sex guy. So she's evaluating the guy much more along the physical lines than even a normal chick during pickup.

Non-monogamy has made me more diligent than the average game guy about diet (no sugar), swimming, lifting, and yoga. Like virtually all people who consciously work to quit sugar, at first the discipline necessary is very hard, but over time habits set in and I eventually stopped missing sugar. I learned to taste real food again and got in the Sunday meal-prep practice to ensure that I wasn't as tempted by easy, quick and horrific foods during the work week.

I'm hardcore about the sugar thing and so hardcore about lifting weights, swimming, and lately yoga because, if you're going to do sex clubs and non-monogamy, the need for good looks and strong sexual skills go up, because chicks aren't much evaluating you, even subconsciously, as a long-term provider guy. It becomes all about the sex.

In the sex clubs, it's also common to strip, pretty quickly, to underwear. She will see you fucking your main girl, too, so she will be able to evaluate your body and sex quality in a very tangible, immediate way. Hot guys with good sex skills get more swap choices.

In contrast, most pickup and online dating is conducted primarily clothed. She can obviously tell some things about your body, but by the time she sees you nude she will probably already have crossed the sex rubicon or gotten close to it. She can also likely tell herself a story about how she can turn you into a provider long term, at least if she really likes you.

Or she's just drunk and horny and doesn't care.

For all humans, though, attraction starts with the body. Just like it does online. Improve your body and you will do better. It is possible for attractive guys in particular to have no game and fail, but it's much less likely.

Bringing women into sex clubs and parties also brings them deeply into a frame outside the mainstream. Some girls will lose their mainstream frame and gain a "sex-positive" frame (you can frame the frame more negatively, if you like). Some will enter that frame temporarily, then go back to conventional frames. Some girls will go wild and then go back to being "good girls" who had a "crazy" youth. Girls who drop in the scene temporarily, with a guy, are very common, and going to sex clubs is not overly compatible with the early stages of family and children: there is too much jealousy, competition, and risk for most couples to make that work. Sex clubs and parties are compatible with the later stages of children and family, though: by the time a couple has been together for six or more years, they're bored of each other in bed. The woman is probably on reliable birth control like an IUD. So the couple often jointly decides to try out sex parties as a way of avoiding affairs and alleviating sexual boredom while still maintaining their primary relationship for the sake of the kids.

Some women obviously don't want kids or have already

had them, and they are often the glue holding a club or a city's scene together. Most women over age 40 aren't objects of intense desire, so their presence or absence isn't as important to players, but some of those women will organize events.

Many younger women can be led into the sex club frame, but as they begin to think long term, they will also fall out of that frame. The diet and lifting help a lot with the initial attraction and dominance parts of the seduction, but for women they're less important for long-term compatibility. Most people, given enough time, almost stop noticing each other's physical attractiveness, which is part of the reason long-term relationships are so hard.

Frequently, a chick I bring into the scene will think about the long-term project, realize I'm not good for that, and we'll break up. Often, it's better if I break up with her or even seed the idea that she should find a father/husband guy who isn't going to be me, no matter what she does. Being honest in this way means that the chick is less likely to do an angry, scorched-earth breakup because she thinks she's been lied to. I don't talk about long-term life goals on second dates, but somewhere in the first year I give chicks my theory of relationships and that helps them decide what to do with or about me.

Many of those girls will leave to pursue a long-term relationship guy. Sometimes the things with that guy works out. Sometimes they don't. When they don't, they will often swing back around to me. I often wish girls good luck when they go. And I mean it. Never emotionally punish a girl who leaves you. Girls are used to guys going to pieces when the girl breaks up: crying, threats, pleadings, begging. When they don't get any of that stuff from me, they're pleasantly surprised, like you are when you get upgraded to first class on a flight.

The smartest, most conscientious women know and understand the gap between fun sex guys and long-term guys. They know the two don't always overlap. And when it comes down to it, they choose the long-term play.

How many women are open to non-monogamy?

Is it 75%? I don't know and it's impossible to say for sure… in a survey done in a cold state for a stranger, I bet only something like 10% of women would be willing to admit they're open to group sex. Of the women I've propositioned for a club or party, about 25% have been eager and excited, about 50% uncertain, and about 25% have been a hard "no," which usually precipitates a breakup because I'm not willing to be monogamous again.

But that's about 75% of the women I've already been sleeping with long enough to ask the question… so it's not a random sample. Chicks who are very reserved, very sex negative, very interested in monogamy, and very unwilling to have pretty quick sex don't like me (and I don't like them). Those kinds of chicks are out there but invisible in pickup writing because they don't respond to street come-ons and online they're very slow-moving. I filter out prudes, though this is not the same thing as filtering out girls who might take some time.

I'm 100% sure that far more women are interested than would admit it in public—or to their boyfriends. Many women who initially say no will come around: first they say no. Then they agree to go to one but do not want to touch or play with others. It slowly amps up. All players are familiar with this… so is any guy who ever dated a girl in high school or just an inexperienced girl. Most chicks won't jump straight into things and need some lead-up and then some processing time.

The most common reaction I've gotten to women who've gone with me to a club or party is, "I never thought I would do that!!!! OMG!!!!" Some experience sub-drop the next day, so care and reassurance is important. Most chicks have no internal feeling gauges so they need a man to reassure and lead them. "Sub drop" is "what happens to your body after you've drained your brain of all the hormones and chemicals that it releases during the scene or session." It a concept most often used by the kink community, but it applies to other areas too. A woman often feels ecstatic when she's in "sub space," or submissive space, being dominated by a powerful man. But when the sex and kink events end, she often drops out of ecstasy, and then "below" her natural or normal state. For that reason, it's important to cuddle and reassure chicks after the event. Always plan to have the chick stay over with you after the sex club or party. As I said, she lacks a man's internal sense of self, so she needs you to reinforce that she's still lovable, worthy, and a good person. If she experiences self-loathing, she will likely fall out of your frame forever.

In a blog comment, the player Nash (currently at http://www.daysofgame.com) said,

> *I can say that most women I've picked up HAVE been to a strip club. Not the same as a sex club, but it's true. And about 50% of girls I've asked are very clear what kind of girl they would pick out at a strip club (that's a fun question to ask a girl).*
>
> *>> Probably if you did a survey, only 10% of women be willing to say that they're open.*
>
> *Mostly… we never care what women say when asked directly. Particularly in a group/public setting. It's more about if you get them in the right mood… what might they say.*

A woman's "truth" changes like the wind. You have to catch her in the right moment to know her potential.

>> I'm 100% sure, however, that far more women are interested than would admit it in public or to their boyfriends.

Another game I play sometimes with women is to talk about 3somes, but turn the question around. I'll tell a girl that most guys have fantasized about being w/ two girls. And then I say, "but most guys don't think much about a girl being w/ two guys." And then, I'll ask if she's ever fantasized about that. Again, hard to say if the answer you get is real...

I'm not into "MMF" 3somes myself, but it's a way to get into the grit of a girls sexual mind.

But this leads me to a similar place in our understanding of women's minds/sexualities... would she like to be DP'd? Would she go to a sex club... and swap partners? The truth is guaranteed to be that this is all more common than most men would expect.

But I think your "women like to follow" comment is very much on point. Without a man to work out logistics and to push for it... the super kinky stuff is less likely to happen.

I'm not a strip club person and think I've only gone with women in tow. Personally, I've found strip clubs expensive and not very gratifying, so once I got into the sex, BDSM, and adjacent worlds I pretty much stopped going. Lots of strippers go to sex positive events anyway, so I can meet them outside of their workplace. I personally would prefer FMF threesomes, like pretty much every straight guy, but I will do both FMF and MFM. More on that in the chapter "Threesome arrangements and management."

* * *

Why do group sex at all? I do it firstly because I think group sex is hot. Secondly I'm not interested in monogamy, probably ever, and I don't think it's practical for most people today. Most people who proclaim that they're monogamists are actually serial monogamists / serial polygamists, so their "monogamy" is only time-limited anyway. Thirdly, lots of chicks really dig it too and they fantasize about it, so let's be cool and make it happen. Fourthly, for players, telling a girl about open relationships and polyamory can allow the player to stay in the game while retaining a girl who would otherwise dump him. Guys worry about "leads to nowhere" and "dates to nowhere." Girls worry about "relationships to nowhere."

I do it for me, for the excitement and the pleasure of the thing. Most people lie about their sex lives and desires. They get frustrated with their partners because their partners are lying too. In my view, sex clubs and non-monogamy short-circuits most of the lying.

If you want to know why people are tuned to lie to themselves, there is a new book, *The Elephant in the Brain: Hidden Motives in Everyday Life*, by Robin Hanson and Kevin Simler, covering it. I'm starting to recommend it to chicks, but of course most chicks are too addled by their smartphones to read a book.

Open or poly relationships from the superior position or inferior position

Red Pill guys routinely slag open and poly relationships because those guys are thinking of themselves as the dude in the relationship with a chick who is going to get laid by a new guy. Or a bunch of new guys. Whatever. While she's doing that, he doesn't have the game to go sleep with new chicks. He might be subsidizing her financially. Those guys say open relationships are just another way for chicks to do hypergamy. It took me a while to understand why the conversations go as they do: the guy is picturing himself financially and emotionally supporting a woman who is laying out new guys all the time. For those guys, sexual scarcity is their biggest problem. They imagine themselves in the inferior position in their relationship.

I, on the other hand, look at open and poly relationships as a possible game tool. I also advocate that men don't marry and don't cohabitate. Marriage is a system for transferring resources from a man to a woman for the sake of raising children, but that system broke down a long time ago for reasons too long to detail right now: a book and website called *Real World Divorce* (http://realworlddivorce.com/) explains why men should not marry today, under almost any circumstance. A legally married guy should never do open or poly.

(Yes, in some ways "open relationships" and "poly relationships" are different, but for players the distinction is irrelevant. It's also true that the word "cuck" has become a general-purpose insult in the Red Pill community, so anyone engaged in any form of open relationships gets called a "cuck" by guys who don't know better and haven't faced the problems that experienced players face.)

For a game-aware guy in the superior position, however, "open" relationships are a handy contrivance to increase sexual availability and keep FWBs or lovers going over the longer term. Sleeping with a chick for a couple months, until she's into you, then taking her to sex clubs or similar venues, and building up the idea of consensual non-monogamy in her mind, can retain her, increase novelty, and make it somewhat easier to sleep with new chicks. But only for guys with good game to start with.

Open or poly is a way to keep her on the rotation while

forestalling her dropping out. The open or poly frame can help make a woman's forebrain align enough with her hindbrain to make her stick around. A guy must make sure a typical woman's primeval hindbrain and recent, reasoning forebrain agree with each other, if she's going to be more than a one-night stand or short fling. The poly system is a way of making her intellectual framework agree with what she is doing sexually. Without that framework, most chicks will eventually dump a guy who won't marry or commit. Almost no one thinks for themselves or questions the society they live in. That applies doubly to chicks, who are creatures of the herd.

At the same time, chicks have lots of naughty fantasies they generally won't share with other people, including, frequently, group sex fantasies—Nancy Friday's books (like *My Secret Garden)*, the success of *50 Shades of Grey*, and the entire romance novel industry show this. Many chicks will act on those fantasies in a given space (spring break, Vegas, bachelorette parties, while drinking) but then deny them to themselves and to others later. Poly is an alternate system that can allow a chick to tell herself that what she's doing is okay and even desirable. A guy who is discreet and non-judgmental can often draw these feelings out of her.

Bi women also make great wingmen.

This superior/inferior situation reminds me of the Nick Krauser post, "Reveal vs Restructure," which describes why some guys think game is pretty simple (just go up and talk to chicks), while some guys find game to be an epic journey on par with Frodo going to Mordor in *The Lord of the Rings*:

So why the divergence in opinion? I think it comes down to which side of this divide you fall on. Is your Journey a process of:

*   *Uncovering a pre-existing [Sexual Market Value]*

SMV and personality that is attractive to women, or;

*   * Ridding yourself of a Pussy Repellent virus and then building an attractive man from scratch?*

The [trainee Chads, who find game relatively simple] are normal men with normal social skills and outlook and inhabit bodies that are reasonably attractive to a wide range of women. Some will require more work than others but all are building on a strong base. It's like cooking a meal starting with fresh organic high quality ingredients. These men already have decent value, they just lack a Value Delivery Mechanism. Teaching them game is like having an out-of-shape teenage Usain Bolt show up on his first day of Learn To Sprint school. They have to put in the work but the rewards are almost immediate. There's never any real struggle.

In contrast, [frustrated chumps, who find game extraordinarily difficult] are a broken mess and the older they are upon discovering game the more traumatic the transformation. Whereas tChad just needs a daygame model and a shove in the back to start opening, fChump needs a complete overhaul of his entire personality and lifestyle.

If you read about game online, this distinction and the endless debates it engenders will be apparent. Guys starting from a very low point have a way different experience than guys starting from a normal point.

"A complete overhaul of his entire personality and lifestyle:" that is a difficult, years-long project. It is worth undertaking, but it is also frustrating to keep working at a project without seeing results.

I bring this up, however, because it parallels a similar distinction among the few who look at open relationships from a game-aware perspective, like myself, as a tool for retention and novelty, versus the more common outlook who see open relationships from the perspective of a guy whose wife, girlfriend, or partner wants to sleep around while he jerks off miserably at home or works to keep a roof over her head. The typical guy knows he likely doesn't have the skill to seduce and sleep with new women, while women interested in casual or semi-casual sex have no problem finding it.

Open relationships fail for most guys because most guys lack the game necessary to make them work. An average guy wants to blind his girl to the other d**k in the world because he rightly fears that if she tastes it, she'll break up with him and swing to someone else. That's why game-aware and Redpill guys online often knock non-monogamy. Open relationships can work for cool guys who are in control, which is a small portion of the male population. They flop for everyone else. Guys who've never been cool and in control HATE open relationships because they imagine themselves as the loser in the open relationship.

Superficially awakened guys who are wildly hostile to open relationships imagine themselves paying for some woman's apartment while she does other guys, rather than the alternate ideal, one in which the guy can sleep around as much as he wants and she will also be his wingman.

Open relationships are also more often discussed in the media today than they used to be; today, practically every women's clickbait website has an article asking if non-monogamy is right for her, so women are primed for it in a way they weren't ten years prior to my writing these sentences. Esther Perel's books and TED talks question the foundations of monogamy and Western marriage. The ideas I'm writing about are percolating through American culture. Feminism has destroyed any reason to marry in the West, save for immigration (I myself have thought about marrying, with a pre-nup, non-American women in order to make sure they can get a Green Card… this is a dangerous and probably stupid thing to do, but I have thought about it). Yet men and women still desire sex, companionship, connection, families —all the things that marriage once bestowed.

Marriage used to be a contract in which men agreed to make money and provide resources to a woman who bears his children and solves his domestic problems. That this contract broke down by the 1960s if not earlier should be obvious.

I want sexual novelty, excitement, and fulfilling relationships. Open relationships can do that, and they can be less atomizing than the relentless hunt that game involves.

Game-aware guys who are open to non-monogamy

The most basic, obvious, important distinction is that guys who know they can get laid have a very different experience from guys who don't. I'm not saying a guy must go out on a random day or night and come back with a chick a few hours later (I can't), but a guy who knows he's got options just has a way different experience and worldview. The options can come from game, ecosystem, doesn't matter, he is just in a different world than a guy who doesn't. ("Scarcity" versus "abundance" are often discussed in these contexts.) A guy is only as good as his options.

I'm not as big a fan of "poly" identification because most people who identify as poly are ugly. Seems to be true of women as well as men. But with an otherwise attractive chick you want to keep on rotation, who might not want to do randoms, saying "poly" and finding another couple or couples to date can work.

Nash, who I quoted earlier, says,

* * *

for me the "poly" community is a fucking mess. I live in California and I am surrounded by these folks… and it's an ugly shitshow. I watch guys "try" this all the time, and they are a fucking sad bunch, mostly.

Can't disagree. That's the average and the median. The worst advocates for poly are poly people themselves.

To me, game, poly, open, motorcycles, online dating, even paying for sex… these are all tools. I'm trying to describe the tools, how they work, how they work for me, how they could work for others, how they are (frequently) mishandled. What tools a guy uses depends on his goals. Most guys flail and fail because they have no tools and have given zero thought to any of this. I don't use all tools all the time. I've not paid for quite a while. That isn't because I'm too good for it or found the Buddha. It's because I've been busy with more conventional pursuits, so I've not needed or wanted it.

Tools can be combined in various ways. Having an incredibly hot girl in a semi-paid relationship who then goes to sex clubs can multiply the effect of both tools (I only recommend thinking about paid relationships for guys who are 35+ and have more income than time. Younger guys should be out working on their game and improving their value, not paying for it).

Game guys have found a great tool. But I think about how some of the other tools fit into game, and how game fits into some of the other tools. Most guys in game don't write much about the other tools. Most guys who like and write about paying for it, don't write about game.

I also don't ask and don't tell. When a recent girl asked me how many partners I've had, I didn't leap forward to say (if she'd pressed I would've said). But I didn't ask her the same question and when I told her I never ask that question of women, I meant it.

Nash doesn't like the idea of bringing a date to a sex club, despite knowing that most girls in uncommitted situations are f**king other guys on the side, and he says,

> *I am being something very close to inconsistent here, but that's the way I am.*

If you're inconsistent and know it, that's okay. I'm a little more worried about people who are wildly inconsistent and don't know it, also known as the entire human population.

When guys talk past each other, it's often good to go a couple levels deeper to try and figure out what is really going on. There may be some deeper synthesis beyond the surface.

Personally, I'm also less moved by pure novelty than some players. Don't get me wrong, I like novelty, but I don't automatically lose interest in a chick after nailing her a couple times. This obviously depends on personality and other factors too.

Poly women are often more masculine and the men more feminine than they should be, so they don't achieve good heterosexual polarity. But I'm still willing to use the poly frame if it matches the girl in question. This works especially well if the girl is a highly attached, bisexual girl who wants to be in a "relationship" with another girl. If she wants to be in a "polyamorous relationship" with another man, I mentally downgrade her to a casual lay and increase my attentions to other women. If *she* thinks we're "poly," though, she'll be happy to keep up the casual sex.

Verbalizing non-monogamy right up front?

"Verbalizing Nonmonogamy Right Up Front" is an interesting post from the writer Blackdragon, who appears to be the only other guy writing about how to incorporate open relationships into game. Blackdragon himself doesn't like telling girls about non-monogamy right up front, but he's published some guys with a different take.

I haven't done online dating for a while, and when I did, I never wrote explicitly about polyamory, as a Blackdragon commenter does:

> *I'm currently [conducting] a strange experiment. Well, it's strange for me, as I'm testing your stuff (going for young hotties on dating sites while being in my late 30s). On my dating profile, I made a little bit of blah blah (nothing interesting, but I write well, so it's ok to have it), but the core of it, the main paragraph states (roughly translated to english):*
>
> *"First of all, I'm polyamorous. I have 2 women in my life, and I have feelings for them. So suck it monogamy!" (very approximate translation)*

I've never tried this. He goes to analyze what might make his strategy work,

> *Makes my profile clearly unique. They contact me because they want to know about polyamory. I'm suddenly not a random profile on the website, I may be the only one stating my polyamorous lifestyle (apart from OkCupid, I don't think many dating sites allow you to show your non-monogamous lifestyle, and OkCupid is not [important] in France).*

This writer has a useful perspective and I'd be curious to hear from more guys attempting the same. His strategy might work. He says that his response rate collapses, *but the few women who do respond are very into him.* To be sure, he's in France, a country with an active swinging scene. When I did online dating, I experimented with a generic "good looking adventure guy" type profile, which usually consisted of one or two activity shots (motorcycle, pools/beaches, that kind of thing), one headshot, one party or group shot, and one or two shirtless pics. Pretty standard online dating things for guys with something going for them. I also experimented with kink and BDSM-themed pics: rope, paddles, cuffs, that kind of thing, in pictures. That also made my response rate decline substantially. That's similar to what commenter Paul experienced:

> *My response rate crumbled to 5% (0% amongst women my age). But two gals contacted me, and showed interest in polyamory as soon as they opened their online mouth (in France, it's not as big as it is in the US). One told me she considers MLTR to be some ideal relationship. The other one just crave for air in monogamous relationships (in my opinion, she should really consider polyamory as a lifestyle).*

When I oriented my online profiles toward implicit BDSM, the big downside I experienced was in terms of quality. A lot of heavy chicks are into kink and BDSM. I don't know if that's because they can't get high-status guys through normal means, or if they're more open about it, or what. I did find some hot chicks through some kink and BDSM-themed pics, but those pics seemed to lock me out of the highest tier of chicks and seemed to suck up some of the lower-tier chicks.

There were fewer flakes, time-wasters, etc. Not zero, but fewer. So I'm not sure what to infer from this. It's also hard to draw conclusions because the online dating world moves so fast. Things that were true ten years ago stopped being true five years ago. Things that were true five years ago may not be true today. For example, I got on Tinder when it was quite new. Maybe in 2012 or 2013? Definitely before it was mainstream. I heard about it from college-age people, and when it first came out I would go to a college campus and get numerous matches. It was like fishing for salmon in a pristine stream. I'd stand by the side of the stream and spear chicks as they swam by. Young chicks who wouldn't touch other online dating systems would try Tinder, "Just for fun." I was older than most guys on it, which worked in my favor among chicks who like older guys.

Eventually I found someone I liked, dated her for a while, and by the time I tried Tinder for real again it was not anything like it had been. Today, it seems like verbalizing non-monogamy in the profile could have interesting consequences, for the reasons the writer lists.

Since I met Libido Girl, pretty much every chick I've been with for a substantial period of time I've introduced or tried to introduce to the sex club scene. I learned to give them the typical books, like *More Than Two* and *The Ethical Slut*. Both books are extremely blue pill and their writers are unaware of key differences between men and women, but they are fine places to start. Most girls get confusing messages about sexuality from their parents and the culture at large. Parents and many cultural products, including religious traditions, emphasize sex negativity, monogamy, and chastity. But many parts of popular culture emphasize that girls just want to have fun, that sexual experimentation is fun, and that everyone is hooking up. Chicks confused and befuddled by the mixed messages they get from their bodies and their cultures. A guy who can read and internalize this book, then share some of its messages with chicks, may straighten out some chicks.

Today there are more chick-friendly books like *Slutever*. Whatever the player uses, it's helpful to try to make the chick's logical forebrain agree with her libidinous, animalistic, hypergamous hindbrain. Chicks also often infer higher status for a guy who is willing to risk losing them through sex with other people. I think chicks wonder, "Why is he not trying to monopolize me, like all the other guys do?" That's a turn-on for most chicks, as they realize the guy has other options.

Two-on-two dating

Most guys are familiar with one-on-one dating. Skills learned in one-on-one dating apply to two-on-two dating, like avoiding politics; searching for common ground; understanding hopes, dreams, and aspirations; listening more than speaking (if possible); having stories to share (if possible); etc. All the stuff from *How to Win Friends and Influence People*, as well as many other books. It's also helpful to gauge the experience level of the other couple: if they're highly experienced, it's easy to accelerate towards sex. If they've never done a "full swap" (the men have sex with each other's woman), go more slowly, take more time, and let them ramp up towards it.

There are two critical parts to two-on-two dating: your girl has to be devoted to being on the same team as you are. In addition, she has to be willing to help you succeed with another couple.

Couple-to-couple dating usually happens when contact details are swapped at a party, or when a couple finds each other online (it's also useful to watch for a guy who tries to get your girl's contact info: if he does, just tell him that you handle dates). If you've met at a party, regular phone numbers or email addresses are typically used. As of this writing, most people online seem to have Kik accounts; people like Kik accounts because they're relatively anonymous, though I'm sure that the company could be subpoenaed for information about the person behind the pseudonym.

Couples from parties are, in me experience, more reliable and less likely to flake, but some will. First dates are not unlike regular first dates, except harder to coordinate, because they require the schedules of four people to mesh, not just two people. They're also more likely to end in sex, if everything goes well.

If your girl is aligned with you, it's useful to carefully evaluate the other couple, even if they already meet your looks threshold. For example, if the guy is a blowhard, or doesn't show reciprocity, or is disrespectful of you, your girl, or his girl, it's time to leave. In normal dates, it's somewhat common for players to fight through some amount of female bad behavior; some bad behavior will be shit tests. On couples dates, bad or indifferent behavior mean it's time to bail. Bad behavior will often be a sign of discord within the couple, or, worse, disrespect for you; the other guy being excited and the other girl being indifferent is common. Some girls will come out on dates at the behest of their primary partner, but if she seems bored or uninterested, it's time to run: she will probably not want actual sex. That's going to be a problem later.

Some guys will also pretend to have a girl, then show up to a couples date alone, saying that his girl is out of town or some other bullshit. When that happens, leave.

Remember the fundamental rule of sex clubs: value-for-value. Guys only bring value if they bring a hot chick with them. In normal, 1:1 dating, "value-for-value" is a little bit different, as the guy is assessing the chick's physical attractiveness and sanity, while the chick is also assessing the guy's physical attractiveness and sanity... but she's also assessing a lot more about his social world, his emotional world, his dominance/prestige, etc. Guys who attempt to "give" too much value in the form of paying for expensive dinners, giving gifts prematurely, etc. are actually demonstrating *lower* value. With 2:2 dating, the value proposition is about two guys bringing two hot chicks to the situation.

There are a fair number of "pic hunters" or "pic collectors" online, and for that reason I'm reluctant to send nudes in advance, in most cases. Sometimes, if the vibe is good, I will.

It's good to think of yourself as a guest in someone else's relationship, and for them to think of themselves as a guest in your relationship. If they don't conduct themselves appropriately, it's time to end the interaction. Interaction problems are especially common among new couples who have no social script to follow, and in new couples it's common for one person to be more excited about non-monogamy than the other person, leading to conflict. That conflict may be submerged at first but will emerge the closer the evening gets to sex. At clubs, I have seen guys start crying the first time they see their partners have sex with someone else, and I've seen the same from women. Most people don't know how they're going to react, which is why doing this while married or cohabitating is so dangerous for novices.

If this seems over-explained, imagine trying to explain conventional dating, in full, both the subtext and context, to someone who's never done it before. The basic idea seems simple, but the complexities are sufficient to fill numerous books (most bad, like *The Rules*) and be the subject of endless gossip. I'm trying to prepare guys for most eventualities.

When I'm doing two-on-two dating, I typically I make minimal effort in that domain. If I'm on the market, I'll give one or two apps or websites a look once a week. Today, Feeld is probably the most common app, followed by OKCupid, but that market is fluid enough that, by the time you read this, my knowledge may be out of date. SwingLifeStyle.com used to be the most common site, but its dated feel dissuades most couples in their 20s. I've heard people discuss SDC.com. At his moment, some other apps or websites may be common; the dating world changes fast enough that what's true today may not be true tomorrow.

It's bad form for opposite-sex individuals to contact one another directly. That is, it's common for guys to talk to each other to make arrangements, for groups of all four people to talk, and for girls to talk to each other, but when a guy contacts the other couple, it's typically for surreptitious one-on-one sex. Players know that, usually, the most difficult time moving a girl to sex is the first time. After the first time, the guy doesn't "count" as a new guy, so the girl is much more pliant. Even guys who can't articulate the situation like this are aware of it, so after a couple-to-couple swap, a fair number of guys will try to arrange secret sex. That's where your girl should tell you, "Hey, Joe just texted me to meet up one-on-one." Then you can either tell Joe to f**k off... or, better yet, you can ask his girl if they're also dating separately. You may find out he's not supposed to be doing that.

This is a game theory problem. In a two-couple, four-person situation, there are strong reasons to defect, for the sake of the sexual novelty. But a hot chick brings automatic value to the situation, so it's bad to let her go sleep with another guy, one-on-one, with no reciprocity.

Two-on-two dating is popular because **it balances the value and reciprocity equations** that destroy couples if they're unbalanced. In a balanced equation, each person in a couple gets sex with someone new; neither has to worry as much about their partner defecting and becoming enamored of a new, third, unknown person. The couple that consciously maintains balanced value and reciprocity is more likely to stay together. See the "Jealousy" chapter for an extended discussion of this idea. It's so important that I'm bringing it up here, as a preview, because players who become manic at the prospect of tons of non-monogamous, uncommitted sex may find themselves leaving their partners behind, leading the partner to become resentful. Women who say they're okay with a guy who can get regular sex with new women are often not really okay with it, when it starts to happens.

A two-on-two date usually gets started in one of two ways: my girl and I match with or contact another couple online, or I collect contact information from another couple at a sex club, a much, or some similar venue. All four of us meet in the same text thread, Kik chat, or Signal group. "All four" is key, particularly when an unknown couple comes from the Internet, because the other "couple" might be a horny guy, and then he messages an hour before the date to say his girl can't make it, but he's still available.

We all chat a little bit. I propose a bar, a date, and a time, coordinating with my girl in advance to make sure our schedules mesh. As with normal online dating, this is often where the other couple goes silent or drops out. If they accept, I try to make sure I have logistics ready for sex, if everyone likes each other: a clean apartment, condoms, good lighting, a hotel (depending on where everyone lives) and the other things guys do to prepare. We meet at a bar. Usually I know within a few minutes whether the other couple has potential, or no potential. If something seems off, I'll usually say, after about 45 minutes, that my girl and I have to go. Most often, it's mutual. Sometimes, the other couple is way less attractive than we are, and desperately wants something to work that will never work.

If everyone seems to like one another, I'll usually get up to go to the bathroom after about forty five minutes, and my girl will do the same. We'll coordinate briefly. If we can't do that easily, I'll sometimes say to the other couple, "Can we have a minute?" We'll move somewhere else, and I'll check with my girl to see whether she wants to bring them home or not. I put zero pressure on her and emphasize to her that, if she's not down, say so, and nothing will happen. If she's a "no," we go back to the table, hang out for a few minutes, thank them for a lovely evening, and leave.

If she's a "yes," I'll often invite them back to my place or to a hotel. Once there, I'll open wine, if possible, and offer it. Ideally, I'll have some gum and such available too. We'll chat for a few minutes. The simplest way to get things started is often to encourage the girls to kiss each other, or to spank each other, or similar. At some point, the girls will often be facing each other, kissing, and I'll be behind my girl, while the other guy is behind his girl. I'll start playing with the other girl's tits, and he'll do the same with mine. Sometimes we'll switch girls then, and that leads organically to the swap. If the other couple are inexperienced, leadership matters, because most girls won't make things happen, and often the other guy is nervous. It's possible to sit on your hands for hours making small talk while sex is on everyone's mind. Don't push hard, don't be a bully, don't be dictator, but do gently suggest activities.

It's also fine to ask the other couple what they have in mind. Experienced couples who don't want to switch will often say things like, "We like having sex in the same room but aren't ready to swap partners on the first date." If the other couple is inexperienced, you can ask if something like that sounds good to them. Same-room sex without swapping is a good way to let the other couple feel out a situation, and then they can decide next time if they want to swap partners.

A common failure mode from two-on-two dating occurs when each guy likes the other girl, and the girls like each other, but one girl doesn't like the other guy (or, sometimes, neither girl likes the other guy). This happens because women are overall pickier than men, and often taken more time to like a guy. 2009 data from OKCupid shows that, in terms of attractiveness, men rate women along a typical bell curve. Women, however, find most men unattractive; as the writer says, "As you can see from the gray line, women rate an incredible 80% of guys as worse-looking than medium. Very harsh. On the other hand, when it comes to actual messaging, women shift their expectations only just slightly ahead of the curve, which is a healthier pattern than guys' pursuing the all-but-unattainable. But with the basic ratings so out-of-whack, the two curves together suggest some strange possibilities for the female thought process, the most salient of which is that the average-looking woman has convinced herself that the vast majority of males aren't good enough for her."

This is probably consistent with the reader's life experience, in which chicks are random, and more picky, than men are. The average man finds the average woman attractive, but the average women doesn't find the average man attractive. Read that sentence twice; that asymmetry powers the two-on-two dating mismatch I'm describing. There are a couple ways to mitigate this tendency.

First, accept that some women are *never* going to be attracted to a given man, in the same way I'm never going to be attracted to a fat chick. Often, there's nothing to be done.

Second, though, "time" and also things like "going to sex parties together" come into play: in every day life, you've probably seen women get into a guy they dislike at first, via exposure. The Mystery rule dictates that the average woman needs 4 – 10 hours around a man to get to sex. Some women need that long, or longer, to decide maybe a guy is attractive after all, and to become habituated to him. A woman might not be attracted to another guy at first, "friends who party together" can work, by increasing the woman's exposure to the guy. The girl isn't into the other guy at first, but we invite the other couple to some parties or clubs. We all do some non-sex things, like get coffee, go to a museum, hit the gym, etc. Over time, the girl starts to like the other guy more, like in normal relationships. First impressions are deceiving. A guy's personality might take time to come out, or to make an impact on the girl. Setting an expectation of "no first-date sex" can let this process happen more organically than it might otherwise.

I'm convinced that a lot of couples who appear to be mismatched in terms of attractiveness, get that way because the two are exposed to each other for an extended period of time—long enough for improbable attraction to develop. There's an online intellectual and sex worker named Aella who made up a "compatibility" quiz for potential suitors; a couple hundred of her pathetic follow-guys filled it out, and she went on a three-day date with one, who she slept with despite not being that into him, and, in her after-action report, she says,

it [the three-day date and sleeping with him] made me really aware of how flexible attraction can be. I wasn't into this guy at all, but with some sustained effort and a few days of close proximity I felt my first stomach butterflies (and I'm now extremely attracted to him). This is crazy to me, and opened up a whole new world – how many other people who aren't attractive to me, could become attractive to me with some effort? This does seem to hold with how other people select their partners, too; proximity has historically been one of the greatest predictors of dating – people you go to church or work or school with. And people falling in love in arranged marriages seems like it might be more the norm than the exception.

* * *

Things didn't work out with the guy, but this is consistent with what I've seen: people at work and school who are neutral at first warming up to each other over time. Girls falling for their teachers makes sense both because the teachers are authority figures and because there's time for those feelings to develop.

Third point regarding regarding women who don't find the other guy attractive: find wanton sluts, the women who are highly likely to be sexually experimental. In the "Stories" section, I describe Ms. Slav and Peaches, two women who fit this category.

Fourth, a lot of guys don't work on themselves. There's a common pattern in long-term couples, in which the girl is more physically attractive than the guy, who's let himself go. His girl loves him for his sense of humor, his providing for her, his being into her and taking care of her, all the rest of that stuff. The new girl, however, wants him to be hot and passionate, doesn't care much about all that other stuff. His dad bod doesn't do it for her. She doesn't care about his job or other achievements. Many guys need to hit the gym, quit sugar, and fix their basic fashion, and more guys than an outsider might think fail to do the basics.

Final topic for this section: flaking. With a typical, one-on-one date, there are only two possible flaking parties. With a two-on-two date, that number increases. Beyond that, many more people are attracted to the idea of consensual non-monogamy than are ready to execute the idea. In many couples, one party will be far more into it than the other, so the one party will get online, create a profile, start chatting, set up dates, etc., only to have the other party veto the whole thing at the last minute.

In addition, some couples like the idea of consensually f**king other people in theory, but when the moment of turning theory into practice arrives, they no longer like it so much. Flaking and ghosting online typically care no consequences, so people are more willing to engage in bad behavior. Expect a lot of flaking in this domain.

When a couple flakes, **I'll sometimes shoot them an email about the next sex club I'm going to and when I'll be there. They can show up, or not**. This might sound like a waste of time to players used to the normal dating world, but sometimes a couple I've interacted with online will show up four or six months later and be down for a great experience. The cost to me is low: I have a list of potential couples on email, kik, and text; I send them the notice before the event or club night; then, if they show up, great; if not, I'm not out much. If the girl is ugly or my girl doesn't like the guy, we can be polite, say hi, and then fade into the background or move on to other couples.

There's one club in particular where I'm somewhat known (and popular) for bringing in newbies, because I'll use the above strategy. Couples can debate among themselves whether they want to show up or not. If they cancel two hours before the date, which is sadly common, my girl and I don't care.

It's not worth taking flaking seriously, and you should assume you'll see more flaking rather than less. I don't spend a lot of time chit-chatting online. After two or three exchanges, I propose a time and place to meet. If they can do it, great. If not, I move on, and I'll keep them around for party invites.

Socializing at sex clubs

I heard from a player who went to a sex club for the first time, and he found about 70 people, most of them decently attractive, yet "there was no one that either of us was 'wow' over (a lot of the girls were still a bit chubby for my taste) but no one was terrible looking" (his girl is very hot, which I want to state for context, and I have seen pics). His experience of the attractiveness level at the club is decently typical... there are not a lot of wow girls, like solid 8s who are 18 - 25, at sex clubs. Some, but they are just not super common, in life or at clubs, though venue and particular night matter as well. If you bring an 8 and another 8 shows up, they will often gravitate to each other, as like finds like. People tend to find others who cluster around their intelligence levels, interests, looks, etc. There are not a lot of true 8s in life, except for guys in the "true 8" age bracket who are in college or some other environment where they cluster. Private groups and parties tend to form, and the hottest people (particularly girls) get invited to them by someone in the know, so they often spend less time in the public venues than less-attractive women.

The other player also found that some people at the club seemed unsure of themselves. That matches my experience, but some couples will appear to keep to themselves because they don't know the social etiquette. Since most other people are scared of approaching, I am often the one who is initiating. Some venues have rules stating that women must approach, etc., but in the real world that means they want guys with decent social skills who aren't cruising. At bad events, socially stupid guys will go from chick to chick, flagrantly hitting on each one and poisoning the atmosphere. We've all seen social morons and what they can do to a party, assuming they don't get kicked out altogether. Think about those guys and how much worse they are at a sex club, and that is why the rules exist. Understand the principle behind the rule and you will understand how the rule can be bent.

Talk guy-to-guy and couple-to-couple, making sure to

include both members of the couple. Don't focus all your energy on girls or you will be "that guy." Encourage your girl to talk to other girls... girls know how to compliment another girl's dress or hair or jewelry. Common conversation topics are whether this is their first time, how they found the club or venue, etc. Really basic openers are fine, like "I saw you two and wanted to come say hi." Even topics like whether they've fantasized about this kind of thing, etc. can work, in the right situation. Normal chitchat about jobs, etc. is also fine... like with normal dates, some normal chitchat that shows you're not a lunatic and some sexual spikes/innuendoes show that you know what's up.

Many people who look closed off don't want to be, so if you can do some normal socializing, you'll ease their mind... there is a popular imagination thing that anyone at a sex club is a crazed sex maniac, and you want to avoid that impression. When you're chatting, you can also do some classic Mystery/Neil Strauss set merges. Talk to one couple, excuse yourself to refresh your drink, talk to another couple, and then introduce couple 1 to couple 2. I am not an expert at this as I'm not naturally the life of the party, but a lot of people will appreciate some social lubrication, even if it is a bit clumsily done (I can be a bit clumsy).

The physical space of a party or club will vary widely: some are essentially undecorated boxes. Some are turned into lush exotic settings. Some of many rooms, some one or two. Some have a single floor, some will have multiple floors. Generalizing about them is challenging; people respond to positive environments, and the better clubs and parties will work to create this environment. Taste and tastefulness is beyond the scope of this book. The better clubs and parties will have a coat check, a bar, this sort of thing. They'll have a warm-up act, like burlesque or dancers. Most often, there'll be a few hours for everyone to chat and meet each other, like a typical cocktail party. Ideally, there'll be some delineation between the sex space and non-sex space.

The initial, chitchat phase phase seeds the possible later switches. I'm more eager to chat with the women who interest me. Women are usually more interested in switching with someone they've interacted with socially, even as little as once or twice, than they are with someone they have never spoken to (this may seem like a small thing to guys, but to a woman even one or two small social interactions can help you break the barrier between her and the outside world... one or two social interactions = this guy isn't crazy = this guy might be safe = this guy is okay to have sex with). Guys who do bar game know that it is often useful to open a woman or her group, then go socialize elsewhere, then re-open her later, because then you will be "known" to her.

For women, much more than for men, sex is an intensely social act. Many more men like anonymous hookups than women. Many men will pay sex workers for anonymous sex acts, and no women will do the same. Even the rare older woman who is paying a man wants that payment to be embedded in a story about her vacation or whatever. At the start of the club night, the party, whatever, demonstrate that you have a little bit of social acuity, that you can make small talk, that you're embedded in a social world and that not a murderous psycho loner of the kind all women have an instinctive aversion to. Will you see some chicks have sex with a man they've never spoken to, once the chick gets into her sex zone? You will. Is that the most regular thing you'll see? No. Make the smarter, higher-percentage moves.

When things start to heat up, you can sometimes invite another couple into the separate sex space, or onto a couch, or wherever, if you like them and you want to access that kind of energy. During the sex itself, the physical space matters... if there is a couple or a woman you're interested in, try to have sex with your girl next to them... then, if you want to trade, the physical proximity is there. Girls will often touch other girls, especially... it's also possible to see if you can touch the other girl a little, just ask first. Sometimes the other couple will say yes (cool), sometimes they will say no (also good feedback). It's common to have sex with your girl, relax for a while, and then switch with another couple for round two.

Like I said, it's a weird environment, especially for people who have never been to parties before or who have only been to one or two. Everyone knows why they're there, and everyone knows that they're going to be f**king in front of each other real soon. The atmosphere is powerfully charged in a way that can be similar to a normal date, when you and the girl know you're heading towards f**king, but it's different when it's in a group.

In non-monogamy relationships that work, "Couples that last put each other first." At parties, smart couples actively work on "putting each other first." They check in with each other. If they have rules, they stick to the rules. You can ask, "What are your rules at parties?" Many couples haven't adequately thought through their rules... if so, it's often better to let them sort out their problems on their own. Often the guy will be more eager to switch than the girl... sometimes the opposite happens.

If you are like me, you want to search for more upscale venues. The downscale venues will be grim, like downscale strip clubs. Downscale strip club are filled with guys who look like they just got on parole and haven't been in civilization in years, and the strippers are so busted I wouldn't upvote them on a dating app.

People who are overweight or underweight or have other problems with lifestyle. Like with everything else, different venues will have different vibes that attract different kinds of people. I'm trying to project a kind of hipster Don Draper vibe, so I want a venue that is going to match that decently. If the venue is off, if the people are off, if anything else feels wrong, leave. If you're an experienced guy at dating and life in general, you should be able to tell the difference between "feels uncomfortable because I'm in a new situation" as against "feels uncomfortable because there is something f**ked up here."

If you like another couple or girl, make a point of taking their numbers later on. You can do this with your phone, but bringing a notepad with you is a pretty good idea because good clubs and parties ban or heavily discourage phones. Arrange couple-to-couple dates, if you and your girl are open to them. Many of the best experiences are in smaller and more intimate settings than the club.

A friend who started conscious non-monogamy this year wrote me to say, "One observation I made of sex parties is that it is one of the few places you can't use your phone. So socializing seems almost old fashioned." He's right: "No phones" seems like a minor thing but it has important implications, because it means that the girls's attention is in the moment, not in the messages that are constantly hitting them. If you are with a girl for a while, tell her to show you her Apple Screen Time app. You will likely be appalled by the hours girls spend on their phones, idly doing nothing. Some guys are just as bad. People at sex clubs and parties are forbidden from using phones for reasons of privacy, so they are actually living in the moment. I wonder if sex parties are becoming more popular because they are one of the few phone-free environments left.

My friend also said, "Honestly, the socializing is a lot of fun as it has an undercurrent of pending sex about it. You also are in a sorting phase where you are looking for connection with couples. I can see why parties are addictive - you can fail at finding someone ... and then they just appear out of nowhere." I've also had this experience.

A typical good party will be an all-night experience: you'll arrive sometime between 8 p.m. and 11 p.m., depending on the venue. Mingle and chat for a few hours. Maybe there will be a show or contest. People will start flirting and making out. If the social space and sex space are formally separated, after one to three hours, people will filter into the sex space and start having sex, and/or swapping partners. Most people go for a round, which may last anywhere from half an hour to an hour and a half, then cool off, go mingle and socialize some more, and then return for round two. Some couples will switch for round two but not round one, and some will do the opposite. I typically want to leave around 1:00 to 2:00 a.m., when I'm fucked out and tired, but some people will stay later. Generalizing is hard. Different parties, though, will have different cultures, so you'll have to judge each party by the party. Some will be very welcoming towards everyone (which can translate to "not an attractive crowd"). Some will be more exclusive (which can translate to "cliquey, and hard to find or get in"). Trying to describe an "average" sex party is like trying to describe an "average" party, since "party" can encapsulate everything from a few teenagers playing video games and drinking club soda to a massive bacchanal of thousands of adults.

Over time, if you're a decent guy who attractive girls like, you'll develop a reputation in the community and then get invites, either solo or as part of a couple, to events and parties. If you're a known quantity, a guy who can bring attractive girls into the scene, you'll be trusted. I've gone to a lot of events on my own, without a date, but those invites happened because I'd been seen with women, and the organizers know that I know how not to be a dumbass. I don't aggressively cruise; I don't flagrantly proposition other guys's dates; I accept "no" for an answer; I read social cues that tell me to get lost. If I'm talking to another couple, I let them do most of the leading and work not to insert myself in their relationship.

Seduction advice encourages assertiveness and aggression in men, and those things have their place, since many guys are overly meek and scared, but at a sex club/party where you're going as a solo guy, too much aggression is out of place—at least during the initial encounter and lead-up.

The consensual group sex scene is also one where speaking counts (as discussed previously in "Verbalizing non-monogamy right up front"). Maybe this is less sexy in some ways than reading a woman's body language and responding wordlessly, as happens in normal dates, but in group situations, or with a woman you've just met, it's dangerous to rely on non-verbal cues; a misread cue will lead to a girl saying you violated her consent, and she'll be right. Better to ask, "Do you want to be spanked?" "Can I kiss you?" etc., rather than thinking that her strong eye contact or coquettish body language speak. As I'm writing this I'm getting ready to go to a friend's party alone, so I'm thinking explicitly about the culture for solo guys who aren't dumbasses.

With all those caveats, some girls *do* want to get f**ked and some couples are looking for MFM, so if you socialize normally and feel there's a possible connection, ask—and be ready for a positive response. A lot of dumb guys are too forward, aggressive, and uncalibrated, but it's also possible to be too meek, retiring, and scared. Women love sex and the types of women who attend a sex party like sex more than normal women.

* * *

I took a few minutes to re-read this section and I find it feels a little autistic, because of the paint-by-numbers, algorithmic description of socializing, but sex clubs are their own little world. This little world doesn't have widely understood social rules, so maybe being super explicit is worthwhile, if strange. It took me a lot of observation to be able to understand what's really going on (the game is arguably just social skills + escalation + looking good + good environment), and it's easy to miss what's really going on. I did, at first. Many of them also have this bullshit equalism rhetoric, which is not really true... the more attractive people are more popular, just like you'd predict, and just like the pretty girls and handsome dudes are more popular. Most chicks are not going to be into guys who they don't perceive as being at least on their level... just like the rest of the world. You can find exceptions, you can be the exception if you are charismatic and have other things going for you, but the principle is universal.

I've learned a lot myself just by trying to articulate the things I think I have learned/discovered. The process of attempting to teach and explain educates not just the reader but the writer. Downside for the writer is of course a lot of unpaid time and effort. But I hadn't thought about all of this until I began to explain what's happening and how the game fits into the sex clubs.

Let me also pause to say this book throws a lot of data and ideas at newcomers. Pull back from the barrage of new ideas and remember not to overthink the experience, despite me dumping a bunch of data. the sex club and party are supposed to be fun and relaxed. If you get too in your head, too into trying to decipher every moment and motivation, the club won't be as fun. Your girl wants to have a fun adventure with you. Think back to high school or whenever you first started dating. If you sweated every detail, every moment, every word said to the girl, you were likely too anxious to achieve flow, and the girl could sense your anxiety. Do enough planning and thinking to make the event happen without driving yourself into over-worry. The first time you try anything new, it's not going to go perfectly. This book distills ten+ years of the game… I have noticed subtleties that won't always be important. Harness the excitement and ride that. Don't let fear be the mind killer.

If you go enough, you'll become part of the scene and community: sex clubs and sex parties will become a lot more fun when you make friends who also regulars and connect with people on a level beyond a purely sexual level. Some of my friends and acquaintances have found employees, employers, business partners, climbing buddies, gym buddies, book clubs, and all manner of other, non-sexual connections through non-monogamy. For most of us, meeting tons of strangers is stressful, and trust doesn't occur immediately upon meeting. It takes time to build, for good reason, since a lot of hours of face time and listening are necessary to evaluate other people (I mention later in the book that players have discovered most women, most of the time, need 4 – 10 hours with a man before sex. Sex clubs can shorten that time, but a lot of swapping happens after two hours of socializing and one hour of people f**king the partner they've brought, getting us close to the four hours many women want prior to sex). As you develop bonds with other people, the clubs and parties will become social *and* sexual events, and they'll be more enjoyable because of those bonds. Like any scene, getting into it will take some time, but ongoing, repeated interactions are more satisfying than one-offs. People who think the sex clubs are purely about sex may be surprised to find that they're as much about socializing, if you're doing them correctly.

Verbalizing sexual escalation in group situations

Players know that most of attraction is sub- or non-verbal, happening through eye contact, proximity, and touch. Most sex clubs have explicit "no touching without consent" rules, for good reason: girls do not want stange men coming up to them and trying to physically intimidate them into sexual encounters. And girls don't want to be involved in one encounter, only to have some other guys try to insert himself in that encounter.

A couple guys have asked how escalation happens. The flirting is fairly normal; with two bi-girls, the guy is there to encourage and facilitate the girls hooking up together. Remember that most girls are used to being pursued, not pursuing, so they frequently need a man to direct the action and encourage them. But with one couple flirting with another couple, things can be more interesting. Typically the two girls will flirt with each other, or the man will flirt with the other woman and vice-versa.

Early in the evening, there will often be flirting, followed by a promise to find each other later. Later in the evening, if sex is already happening, it's common to invite the other couple to the playroom or sex area. If the other couple agree, they're interested. On two-on-two dates, just invite them back to your place.

Once you're in the sex area or your own apartment, there are two main points where words come into play: "Can I kiss you?" and "I'm going to get a condom" or "Should I get a condom?" I like "I'm going to get a condom" with eye contact; it gives a different default path than the question route. Verbalizing is important here because it means the girl is less likely to go "OMG non-consent!!!!!", and verbal consent also harmonizes expectations. You know what to expect. She knows what to expect. Your girl knows. Her date knows. If this is happening couple-to-couple, I'll look to her for agreement. Then I'll look to her date and make sure he agrees well. If he nods or says okay, I'll proceed. Often, I'll encourage the two girls to kiss first, then start kissing the necks of one of them. Most girls have never been kissed by two or three people at once and love it.

Reputation is paramount, so you're better off dropping one flakey lay than producing drama or f**king up your reputation through poorly defined agreements. In regular dating, guys know that a lot of girls like drama and like testing men through last-minute resistant (LMR), which should be overcome through persistence or freeze outs. Not so here, in this world. Take a raincheck, exchange numbers later, and arrange a later date. You don't want girls going around saying, "It wasn't my fault, he just made me do it!" You don't want her to have a problem with her boyfriend or husband later. Girls love to avoid responsibility for their actions, and for a lot of girls the feeling in the moment is everything. If a girl feels the next day that she has been taken advantage of, she will forget her in the moment "yes" and then tell herself and maybe others that she was abused. Men may argue this is irrational, but I'm describing the process, not making an argument for rationality.

While skilled players often work with this fact in one-on-one situations, groups are a different game that require superior calibration. Recriminations between couples can happen if one part of the couple outpaces the other party, and girls are prone to next-day regrets, particularly if they say yes reluctantly.

If the girls have been kissing each other for a while, I'll kiss the other girl, while the other guy kisses my girl. The escalation here proceeds pretty normally, until you mention the condom. If the new girl is hesitant or not really into the makeout or the touching, pull back, say you understand, and re-engage with your girl. Tell your girl, "Hey, Madison here doesn't go further, so perhaps we should all back off this." If the girl isn't fully engaged, you want to avoid a situation in which the other guy is railing your girl, while his girl gets cold feet and says no. To avoid this situation, everyone should be escalating at approximately the same rate. You also want to avoid rooting a pretty and eager girl, only to have her date angry or sad because he's not ready for the swap.

If everyone is not on the same page, don't be afraid to encourage your girl to stop. If she won't stop, she's not your girl anymore. This hasn't really happened to me too much. I've usually explained reciprocity and fairness to the girls I bring, and that prevents most problems. Ms. Slav, a current partner as I write this and who is discussed in the "Stories" section, has not always played by those rules, which has created some problems and led me to downgrade her. She's an exception, because most girls will follow your lead. Most girls also understand that, if the other girl isn't ready for sex, she shouldn't have sex with a strange guy.

Sometimes the other girl will be down for sex and the guy won't be. Same ideas apply. If one party in another couple is gung ho and the other party isn't, grab your date and bring her out of the space for a bit, if that is a reasonable thing to do.

A typical, smooth encounter moves from flirting, to the girls kissing, to the girls kissing the other guys, to clothes coming off, to sex. Maybe with some BDSM in between. It's often useful to ask the girl if she wants to be spanked or paddled, as that is a good intermediate space for her to get in the zone.

With the "Can I kiss you?" question and the "I'm getting a condom statement," affirmed by all present, there are no problems in the moment. Players are familiar with one-on-one escalation, and, if you are not, a book like *The Sex God Method* or *She Comes First* will help you there.

Jealousy

Nash says:
> *I would be interested in jealousy. I'd like to hear not only "it can be avoided," but some EXAMPLES of how it has come up, show both sides, and then your best practices, some case studies of how you've managed that in YOURSELF and the GIRLS.*

I don't think jealousy can be wholly avoided, for most guys. It's like pain in the gym: you're going to feel it sometimes. Most guys, including me, don't like to see other guys railing their chick, even if the guy and chick are dating casually. Some amount of jealousy, however small, arises in couples because jealousy is adaptive. Jealous guys have, historically, been more likely to ensure that a chick is bearing his child and not some other guy's. The vast, overwhelming majority of human existence occurred before reliable contraceptives and DNA tests. We are not going to overcome our evolved instincts to do "mate guarding" (the term evolutionary biologists use). Not perfectly. This excerpt, from *The Ape That Understood the Universe: How the Mind and Culture Evolve*, further describes jealousy from an evolutionary perspective:

Throughout the course of our evolution, any trait that increased the chances that a man would end up investing in his own offspring, rather than the offspring of his good-looking next-door-neighbor, had a good chance of being selected. One such trait was jealousy – the kind of jealousy that would lead a man to keep a wary eye on his partner and the good-looking neighbor, and to do what he could to keep them apart.

For most guys, jealousy can't be avoided because we've evolved to feel jealousy and be hypocrites. So if a guy wants to go down this path, he has to know that **some amount of jealousy is probably coming** and be psychologically prepared to experience it, before it happens. A guy can rationally understand that he's doing a quid pro quo: he's going to get his, so she's going to get hers. This helps, but the jealous response is more emotional than rational. It is very hard to overcome an emotional response through rational thoughts, but it can be done and for many guys must be done.

If a guy is in a casual relationship, he knows (intellectually) that the girl is probably sleeping with other dudes. He also probably likes the deliberate ambiguity, the way he doesn't ask her and she doesn't tell him. So he can think to himself, "Maybe she's only having sex with me," while he knows… that's probably untrue. How big a jump is it from knowing that intuitively to seeing it happen in front of you? A big one, emotionally, but a small one, intellectually, particularly if the guy is busy with another chick.

In addition, I deal with jealousy by focusing on the other chick. Libido Girl, who properly introduced me to this world, made sure that I was having sex with another girl before she had sex with another guy. Smart girl. It is hard to get that angry while you are deep in another girl. Libido Girl did check in with me after all four of us were done having sex, to see how I felt, and again later that night, and again the next morning. She was helping me to emotionally process what had happened.

Now I do something similar with most girls I'm introducing. I encourage them to go first, or for us to go concurrently. Often, we don't have sex with other people on her first night at the sex club. I try to get them involved somewhat gradually, unless they are very gung ho, like Ms. Slav.

Jealousy can be better overcome when you (the man) and your date agree to only bang other chicks together, or to only do a couple-to-couple swap. You don't want her entering a threeway with another couple on her own volition, leaving you abandoned.

Jealousy goes away over time, or a guy becomes acclimated to it. The first time a guy brings a date to his party, jealousy may be overwhelming. But as one becomes acclimated, it decreases; if someone is desperately scared of flying, a psychologist won't get her on a plane right away. A psychologist will gradually ramp her up (first he'll have her in a plane-like dwelling, then talk to her about it, etc.). Jealousy can be the same way. Today it's normal for me to have sex in groups or trade couple-to-couple, so much of the jealous response is gone.

The other way I see people deal with jealousy is, realistically, boredom. Many couples have been together so long that they aren't that sexually hot for each other anymore. For those guys, jealousy can be a bit useful, because it might make him want to "compete" for the woman he's tired of listening to every day. Couples who have been together so long that they're bored may feel less jealousy and, when they do feel jealousy, it may help them.

Another word about swapping: Guys who don't want their chick to bang other guys are in for problems. If the chick is bisexual, she may be okay with seeking another woman. The unicorn path is not impossible but it is also the route of much drama and nonsense. I'm not going to speak to it here because the reader can search for "unicorns and swingers" or "how do I find a unicorn" and read the endless shit written about this overdone topic.

To summarize, I don't think there's a single cure for jealousy because jealousy is evolutionarily adaptive. Jealousy can be overcome by applying rational thinking to an emotional sphere, which has its own problems (I'm aware of them). It can also be overcome by the guy focusing on his own experiences: when you're in another chick, who has the energy to feel jealous? These methods are imperfect and there is no final "right" answer. That is why everyone discussing swinging, open relationships, and polyamory online discusses jealousy. If there were a simple solution, everyone interested would do it, ending the discussions. But there is no simple, one-size-fits-all solution, so it's probably the most-discussed topic in non-monogamy. Many people dream about a mate who is loyal while allowing his or her partner to screw around.

Given how most players like sexual novelty and variety, and most women in uncommitted relationships are going to be f**king around anyway, a guy should think about some of non-monogamy as a way of achieving better output for less work while also retaining the girl better.

It's also surprising to me that more players haven't figured this out. Maybe I'm lazier than some players and like having some of the filtering work done for me, in advance.

A few guys are also into jealousy. Jealousy makes them angry and competitive and then makes the sex better, because they want to do better than the other guy, or reclaim "their woman" and that kind of thing. These guys cite the Robin Baker book *Sperm Wars* and use the word "compersion." That is not my experience but if this is you, great.

* * *

Jealousy is often most acute when your partner isn't in the same room; someone who is happy to have sex with lots of different people often doesn't really truly want their partners to do the same. But it can be easier to handle the jealousy if both parties are getting the same thing at the same time in the same place.

One player, Black Ring, had a woman who has spent most of her life being very promiscuous and hoping from man to man (and woman to woman: she's bisexual). He introduced her to sex clubs and gave her a framework for placing and thinking about her non-monogamy. She went out and f**ked a couple new guys. Then, when he did something similar with women, she couldn't handle it. She seems to not have realized that Black Ring is a guy who can seduce new women, and when he did, she flipped, and broke it off with him. Eventually he reeled her back in, but he expected that she would be okay with him doing the equivalent of what she was doing. She's a hypocrite. Many of us are.

To be sure, Black Ring likely didn't manage the woman optimally. As a couple, they jumped too deeply into non-monogamy too quickly. Both also had other obligations specific to their individual lives that may have prevented deepening their relationship first. They should have gone more slowly, with her agreeing not to f**k random other guys, and both of them focusing more on the sex club and dating environments. Instead, she wrote checks she couldn't cash, claiming that she would be fine with him having sex with other women.

Black Ring didn't blame her; instead he thought about how he can do better next time. At work, the wise manager tries to internalize as much negative performance from his subordinates as possible. He asks himself how he could have handled the situation better, how he can handle it better next time, etc. The bad manager blames his subordinates, to maintain his own mental image of himself. Sometimes the good manager gets bad subordinates and sometimes the bad manager gets good subordinates, but the best managers conscientiously try to prevent bad situations and encourage all subordinates to do the best work possible.

When you're introducing a woman to non-monogamy, encouraging her to only have sex with others with you is a good strategy that is more stable than most other strategies. Moving slowly is a better way to manage emotions than moving quickly. I want to emphasize that you, as a player, can pursue relationship anarchy and win. It's possible for you to move quickly into non-monogamy and win. The relationship is just less likely to function that way, and more likely to blow up, if you dive in quickly and don't work hard on jealousy management and mitigation strategies, like the ones I've mentioned about dating other couples, equality and balance, etc. I'm speaking in probabilities, not absolutes.

I've never heard anyone say, "We got into non-monogamy or sex clubs too slowly." The reverse, however, is very common: people leap in too quickly, then create emotional explosions that destroy their relationships. So going slowly is often better.

Lifting offers another metaphor: many guys, particularly older guys age 30 and over, hit the gym too hard and too soon, and often don't have good enough warm-ups and mobility to lift the kind of weight they want to lift. Rapidly adding weight to the squat, deadlift, clean and jerk, overhead press, and bench press is a good way to hurt yourself and ultimately retard your progress. For guys who aren't targeting peak strength at a particular date for a contest, like basketball playoffs, it's better to go a little slower. Guys who are being coached for peak strength at a specific section of a sport season or wrestling match have different needs and should consult their coaches. Guys who are starting a workout program for fitness, aesthetics, and improved bodily functioning should add weight a bit more slowly than they think, and avoid injury.

I've seen a lot of failure in this world, and seeing all that failure results in the caution expressed in this section.

One other interesting thing: in couple-to-couple dating online, it is very useful to have an array of sex pics and short videos available. They're a system of "proof" of sorts. In normal online dating, sending a single chick a sex pic or video will immediately end the interaction. In couple-to-couple dating, it is more common and gets closer to "proof" that the guy is desired by other women. I do this part very well. There are single guys who are just seeking dirty pics, so they have to be avoided, but the picture-proof is there.

Threesome arrangements and management

Some people think threesomes "just happen" and while some threesomes can, guys who do non-monogamy look for the principles and patterns underlying threesomes (besides drugs and circumstance... not my favorite routes). The biggest principles are the ones you're already thinking about because of reading this book: reciprocity and bringing value. In an MFM threesome, the value can come from just being able to set up and execute the scene... lots of women have MFM fantasies but find them very hard to bring to fruition, since most guys are very touchy about this topic and afraid of losing their one and only girl. In many couples, there will be an agreement to do an FMF, then do an MFM, but one person will be eager to do the threesome that is in their favor then don't want to reciprocate, leading to the usual hurt feelings, drama, cries of double standards and hypocrisy, etc. Girls are very used to guys eager for FMF but who won't seriously entertain MFM.

Where there is a shortage there is an opportunity, and smart guys ruthlessly exploit sexual marketplace arbitrage opportunties. A shortage of guys who will fulfill a woman's fantasy means higher value for a guy who can.

My friend "John" has played the "threesome buddy" role for me, and me for him. We don't really keep score (no point), although I think we are both transitioning out of this space and into other roles. Many guys will take a free lay but not reciprocate; John reciprocates, which is good, because if a girl confesses her MFM threesome fantasy, I can say, "If you are serious about making it happen then we can make it happen." All three of us arrange a time to get a drink and make it happen.

We meet in a bar, and either I set the expectation with my girl or the other guy does with his. If the girl is mine I tell her that she can back out any time for any reason. Chicks need an open, low-pressure environment to really enjoy the buildup, and to make sure they can exercise mate choice. At some point in the evening, when the other guy goes to the bathroom, I check in for a thumbs-up or thumbs-down. If I'm with another couple, I'll strategically go to the bathroom for a few minutes or run out to "take a quick call" to give the couple a chance to talk.

It's also possible to do a genuine hour-long meetup, then have the threesome at a later time after the chick has had time to process who I am, or who the other guy is. Not being in a rush lets women feel comfortable. If it's a go, I like to have restraints, a paddle/flogger, a blindfold, and a couple other relevant toys for the situation. Like nipple clamps or clothespins. Those depend a lot on the girl's sensitivity and should only be used when checking with her.

At the private space, to begin the process, I will let the girl get accustomed to the new space and environment for a few minutes, as with a typical bounceback. I'll put on music and adjust lights as needed. Often there is a weird energy in the room, and the conversation will move to very non-sexual prattle that kind of denies why we are all here. People feel weird about being the "one to start," unless they have done this before and integrated it into their personality. After five or ten minutes, I will often start.

If the girl is sitting I'll tell her to stand up. The other guy and I will kiss different parts of her neck. The best way to make it happen is usually one guy standing in front of her and the other guy behind her. Girls report that four hands and two sets of lips on their bodies is amazing, and it yields sensations not possible with only one other person. I try to make sure everyone is included to the extent possible. Gradually the girl's clothes come off, and I will undress myself or let the girl undress me, depending on what's happening. Sometimes I will spank her and bend her over and paddle her for a while. Depends on the energy. Foreplay is more straightforward than you might think. When it's time I often bend a girl over the corner of a bed and take her from behind and have her fellate the other guy, because I prefer the girl's p***y. Sometimes I won't get hard immediately because the atmosphere can be super stimulating. Not worrying about that is key to overcoming it. Some girls like to have two c**ks to suck, one in each hand, swiveling from one to the other.

Then it's kind of a free-for-all that varies by girl and circumstance. After the first nuts have been had by all, sometimes I will get out massage oil.

For FFM, the overall process is similar, except girls are much flakier. Most often I am with one girl more than the other, and my girl and I act as a team on the other girl. The drink and date are similar. Sometimes I will try and get the girls to kiss each other at the bar. At the private space, sometimes I will have the girls take turns spanking each other. When the time comes, sometimes I will f**k one girl while she goes down on another. This is fun but not a good way to let the girls orgasm, because most women need very specific rhythms for an extended period of time, so most often there will be periods of one on one with the third party assisting or watching.

More rarely, I meet a girl who right away confesses her MFM fantasy. If she is a sex maniac met off an app or through similar means, I like having the threesome ready to go, with my friend John; if you get into the non-monogamy scene, you may "borrow" a guy from a couple… which can be a turn-on for the guy's girl, because she knows other women want to f**k him. For a sex maniac girl, the MFM may be a long-term fantasy she's never achieved.

In date terms, sex maniacs are different than normal girls and the risk of NOT f**king her is greater than the risk of f**king her. With normal girls, there is a risk of "overcooking" her and then setting off her anti-slut defense (ASD), which players know about. With a girl who is heavily into being sex-positive, non-monogamy, BDSM, etc., there is a risk that she has an overfilled schedule and really wants to get f**ked, so if you don't f**k her, she will be unsatisfied and go home and start texting whoever else she has available for sex. If she's good looking she'll find someone.

MFM has one other subtle, but important point that I have never read or heard explicitly stated: it can be a tool for keeping the girl at an emotional/relationship distance. "What?" you say, "Don't you WANT the girl to be in your orbit and frame?" Well, maybe. Guys who have never had a girl invest in them will be obsessed with getting quality girl investment for the first time. Guys can have a different problem, though…. the girl invests and wants a relationship. Guy says no. Girl leaves. If you listen to chicks, they complain about "f**k boys" (happened to me a couple months ago) guys who are "just players," guys who are "assholes who break my heart," etc. This talk is mostly sexual market value mismatch, and she's getting these problems because she's pursuing guys +1 or more above her… when there are plenty of guys at or below her level who would be *thrilled* to commit to her. She doesn't perceive this way however. If she consistently has sex with one guy, she'll end up in love with him and wanting a relationship. A player who wants to f**k many women will have to negotiate this problem, or pattern, many times. MFM may keep her from rapidly pursuing a conventional relationship.

If she's f**king other guys, even with you, she may stay at that emotional remove. She may not bond with you the way she might if she is orgasming only from being railed by you. If you don't want that…. this could keep her at bay. Paradoxically, it can also make her closer to you by making you the one guy who can fulfill her fantasies. You're extending the range of possibility with semi-regular MFM. Which way it goes… depends on her, and on you.

Subconsciously most men want to monopolize women because letting another cock near her creates paternity uncertainty. In a world without birth control that's a decent way to make her try to finger you as the daddy when you might not be. Our psychologies remain in the stone age even as we know that she's coiled up with an IUD and crotch fruit is unlikely. Most of us are controlled but our subconscious impulses far more than we want to admit. This is also why tribal politics are so dumb most of the time… most people want to see their team win. The same right-leaning people who are rooting for a shameless grifter would be howling with outrage at a left-leaning politician doing one-tenth of the same shit. Tomorrow it will all be reversed.

I get away from the point… writing all this out has been interesting. Have I become group-sex Jesus? I have been hearing from guys who have read my work and are trying out the techniques. I am encouraging some to write field reports and a couple are said to be in progress. If (when?) they come in, I will post the results, good or bad.

It's easy for threesomes to fall apart for all kinds of reasons, but making this kind of special experience happen for a woman who has wanted to do it, but in a safe and controlled setting, can be powerful.

I don't think many threesomes happen when a guy meets two new women who already know each other. In an FMF threesome, the girls are the limited factor and the guy is the common factor. Two girls who already know each other don't need a guy to get them to hookup. If they do, almost any guy will be fine. These kinds of threesomes seem to happen most often when a guy and a girl consciously (or unconsciously, when drunks) decide to seek or seduce a third girl.

Clearly it's possible to do a threesome with two girls who already know each other, but I don't think that pattern is as common as other patterns.

There is no easy way

Being a player is hard. Most guys must churn constantly for new leads. Old leads drop off. Chicks are of course flakey, because they're testing for a guy's quality. Neither online nor offline dating is fast for most guys. The economic conditions that make game plausible have only existed in the West for a couple decades.

Being in a monogamous relationship is hard. Sexual boredom will likely arrive, no matter how hot the sex is at the beginning. Romantic attachment will replace passionate attachment. Most chicks expect financial subsidies in a monogamous relationship and will seek guys who provide those subsidies. Most chicks want kids if they don't have them already. Worse still, some chicks will already have kids and be looking for a new guy.

Being in a non-monogamous, hedonistic relationship is hard. One needs all of the skills of the general player, and one needs the personal temperament to want to do non-monogamy. The player needs to re-wire the chick's internal psychology to make non-monogamy a part of the chick's identity and toolkit. Not all chicks will go for it.

Gathering enough information to make rational decisions about the world is hard. One needs a lot of practice in the real world as well as a lot of reading and networking with other players to understand the world. Dominant information sources are not helpful for most aspiring players. Many are inaccurate or written from a woman's perspective. Even sources of information that are better-than-average, are often not the best.

Discipline is hard. That's true in terms of diet, mind, information diet, and body. It's true in terms of work. Discipline is one reason I was reluctant to write online for a very long time.

While the above paragraphs are true about the individual guy, every guy is simultaneously doing his thing to try and get laid:

- The military guy is being a tough badass to make chicks think he'll protect them and that he's competent.
- The music guy is literally seducing chicks with the

sound of his music.

- The athlete guy is expressing his physical fitness and his ability to dominate other men.
- The business guy is demonstrating the quality of his mind and his ability to outcompete other men in the industry. He's demonstrating his capacity to support a woman and provide a good home for her and her children.
- The professor is demonstrating intellectual mastery and also has a natural leadership position over the students in his class.
- The laid-back surfer and weed guy is demonstrating how chill he is and how a girl can relax and focus on pleasure with him.

There are many others.

A guy can only embrace his version of the hard way. I have it easier than many guys but also harder than a lot of guys. My way has been hard and remains hard to this day. The hard path is an essential component to life. When I was younger I thought I could find "the easy way" with women. But there is no final, easy way. There are ways that are more or less relevant to a given guy, but none is easy. To succeed, a guy should embrace the pain. The pain of learning. The pain of working longer and harder than other guys. The pain of creating when others merely consume. The pain of being John Galt.

To me, the non-monogamous way is easier, better, and more plausible than some other alternatives, but "easier" is still hard, and it still has to suit a guy's personality. This way suits my personality, though may not suit yours.

There will always be a relative shortage of hot chicks in the hottest age range (just as there is always a shortage of top guys, from a woman's perspective). Guys from the onset of puberty to the onset of senescence will always be competing for the relatively small number of hot chicks age 18 – 30 (sometimes 35). Game and evolutionary biology will clarify female psychology, but it's still necessary to execute effectively. Most guys cannot or will not. Player blogs are typically written by the rare guys who go, or are going, the distance.

Attention is the only tool modern men have

"Let's say a girl is acting bitchy," is a good essay:

> *When having a boundary crossed actually means you'll walk out, and you have zero tolerance for bullshit, it will show up as soon as the micro transgressions happen. This permeates the whole thing since your very first moment.*

The only real tool modern men have at their disposal is attention. You either give attention or withdraw it. That's really it. The rest is commentary. When you blow up a girl's phone you're dissipating one of the only (or the only) tool(s) you have.

There is a wonderful book by David Barash, *Out of Eden: The Surprising Consequences of Polygamy,* that lists all the tools men used to have to enforce monogamy. They could kill their wife's lover (seriously, that used to be legal in the United States). They had physical force. They had the weight of society enforcing monogamy. Abandoned women would face big, serious consequences, unlike today, when most women leave the moment they think they can get a better guy. Women are supported by the government in the form of the welfare state and will go to the government to take a man's money from him.

Now, in the contemporary world, men have nothing but

attention itself, which is one of many reasons why marriage is such a bad deal for men, at least in the United States. Attention is the only resource men have.

This is also why I think most men should not use most social media. Social media gives women attention and validation that is unlikely to lead to sex. A woman loves attention almost as much as a man loves sex.

It's not impossible to use social media well, but it's never or pretty much never a good idea to "like" women's photos and statuses—yet I see guys do this all the time. As more people primarily exist in the (fake) digital space, guys who can drive interactions in the real world will become more and more valuable.

When a woman crosses a boundary, withdraw attention. Better yet, give attention to other, better behaved women. Guys with options are very different than guys without. Girls know you have options when you shut the fuck up. "Shutting the fuck up" is a rare skill in today's verbal diarrhea culture.

Chicks also know you're high value when you stop giving them attention and start directing your attention in the only places you should: your skills, your life, the women who are having actual sex with you.

In non-monogamy, you'll run into many people online who like verbal attention but have no real interest in meeting up. They should be cut off. If a couple decline three meeting offers, move on, or only invite them to parties or events. If a man or couple waste their attention, they're displaying low value, and that will haunt them throughout their time in the non-monogamy scene.

Non-monogamy is sufficiently unusual that almost every city will have a distinct "scene" with particular players in it. Most scenes probably have fewer than 1,000 regular people in them. Some will drop in and drop out. Your reputation in this scene will likely come to matter, and for that reason it isn't a good idea to castigate other couples, for the same reason there is rarely any reason to give girls verbal lashings. Those lashings just make girls withdraw and generally don't advance the man's interest. They may feel good in the moment but hurt a man's inner game and reduce his long-term prospects.

The book *Games People Play* by Eric Berne is also about attention and managing relationships. It's also recommended. It won't teach you how to open, stack, and vibe with a chick, but it will help you analyze what is really happening in human relationships.

People get dissatisfied with what they have

People who are in very long-term relationships get bored of their partner and eventually crave something new, different, or novel. That's why Esther Perel's books are best-sellers: she admits and describes what many people feel.

The other part of the relationship theory is that people who are always having short-term relationships and experiences eventually feel anomie, loneliness, existential meaninglessness, and a longing for deeper connection to another human being.

I don't see a way of resolving the tension between long-term comfort (and its concomitant boredom) and short-term excitement (and its concomitant loneliness). The long-term players I read (Krauser, Tom Torero, etc.) make me wonder if they really are going to be picking up girls forever—in another decade, are they still going to be stopping a girl to say that she looks like a greyhound, or like she just got out of yoga but didn't have time to change?

Maybe the answer is yes. Some artists practice their art until their deaths. I will not argue that PUAs are eventually going to recant and shack up. Neil Strauss famously did this and wrote *The Truth*, about it but has since filed for divorce, so maybe he's back to being a player. I see most couples eventually tiring of each other and descending into squabbling, and I see most singles tiring of the dating grind and the Groundhog Day effect of casual sex. Some who marry and want to keep their relationships fresh turn to sex parties as a way to create novelty and alleviate boredom while still maintaining their comfortable bonds with one another. This kind of solution can go sideways, but for some people it seems to work.

I begin to think that humans are by our nature discontent, and there is no final answer.

But I don't know how a person lays out a life or plans well for the future that way.

For a long time I've been a sex-positive, sex-is-the-center-of-life person. *Cheap Sex* by Mark Regnerus lays out many of the downsides of the sex-for-all, all-the-time culture that I believe in. He is wrong or at least misguided about some things, like the way he underemphasizes the extent to which modern sex and dating is driven by women's desires to date and marry "up." Women who consciously stop playing that game find a guy and get married. Women who feel the need to always move up, often don't marry. They end up alone.

But his chapter on "The Genital Life" makes me think, maybe there is something hollow about what I've been doing. Maybe like everything, done long enough, it gets boring eventually.

It's telling that almost all the online PUAs who write books and keep blogs had a substandard high school, college, and early 20s experience. Just like Neil Strauss. Maybe guys do eventually work it out of their system. I'm not saying that I think tagging new chicks is bad. I still get that thrill. But afterwards, now, I more often get the, "Is that it?" feeling.

And it is more of a feeling than a verbal question. The answer might be "yes," and I have to focus on the positive. Most guys never achieve game skills or abundance: getting to that point is amazing and I'm blessed for it.

The question is… what's next? What then?

Maybe I know too much for long-term relationships. Knowledge can poison. For most guys, the answer is likely children.

Game starts with concrete skills and ends with philosophy.

The downsides

The obvious downsides to non-monogamy are alienation of affection and paternity uncertainty. The former is an inherent risk in modern relationships. The latter can be ameliorated but not eliminated.

It's conceivable, of course, that a chick will get pregnant and not know who the baby daddy is, and for that reason DNA testing is normal in the non-monogamy community. These problems seem pretty uncommon, because most chicks in the scene have IUDs or have found hormonal birth control that doesn't mess with their libido.

There are still other problems; these can be seen as common failure modes for non-monogamy.

- If a guy is hunting the hottest girls, the ones who are 8+, he is not likely to find them, or find many of them. I have seen some, but they are rare and in high demand. If a guy brings high 7s and 8+ girls, however, he will be the king of his local scene (I have played this game very successfully). In the United States, very few chicks remain solid 8s or higher past age 25 or 26. Most chicks eat too much sugar and too many simple carbs to stay at that high level. I have met exceptions to that rule, but not many.

- A guy still needs to find a compatible woman. This version of lifestyle or ecosystem must be layered onto existing game for it to work. Chicks are flakey by nature, which often makes them ill-suited to high-level corporate jobs, and attempting to introduce them to non-monogamy will increase flaking.

- A guy will be evaluated very directly based on his body and sex skills. If either are lacking, everyone will know it because everyone will see the guy nude and f**king. Because (almost) everyone gets naked and has sex at these clubs and parties, I have an unusual amount of experience in evaluating how chicks look clothed and unclothed. Many chicks who seem one way clothed turn out another way when not.

- You may lose your girl, or some girls. Girls enter into the reality of any guy who f**ks them good. Girls lose the excitement and novelty of one guy when they f**k another. A girl may become infatuated with a guy she meets at a party who she connects with, then swing away from you and to him. This isn't incredibly common, but it has happened to me and it is a real risk. On the other hand, a girl who is open to experience and likes trying new things will sometimes bond *more* closely to the guy who brings her into the scene. He is the guy who fulfills her fantasies and understands that she has a lot of love to give but also doesn't want to be 100% monogamous.

- Some chicks will be disgusted by the concept of group sex and dump you straightaway. This isn't terribly common if you've brought the chick deeply into your world, but it does happen. If she wants your baby, and you're like "Let's go f**k other people

together," she has a very clear sign that you're not a
  suitable long-term choice for providing financial
  subsidy.

- Normal parties will become boring. I had a
  conversation with "Bike Girl" that went like this:

"My friend is having a New Year's party. Maybe we should
go to that instead."

"Have you been to his parties before?"

"Yeah."

"What's it like?"

"It's fun."

"Is it a dozen people standing around drinking and
awkwardly eyeing each other up, only to have none of them
go home with each other at the end?"

"Haha."

"Like I said, we can go to the sex party, where instead of
people wondering what everyone looks like naked, they can
find out for themselves. You've liked the things we've gone
to, right?"

"Um, yeah."

"Right. So I have to give them money towards the hotel, so
if we're going to agree to do this, we need to do this."

"Okay. I feel bad because usually I hang out with [the
usual friends.]"

"That's okay. I don't think your friends are down for this,
but 'Melissa' might be. You can talk to her about it if you
want."

"Haha, okay."

Normal parties that consist of basic people getting drunk and
making small talk are boring. They're only exciting to the
extent two people are attracted to each other and want to go
off to f**k. Usually, you'll know if this is a possibility within

half an hour to an hour of arriving. I can't even tell you how many boring parties I've wasted my life at.

There are some other common forms of bad behavior:

- A man and woman create some set of rules for playing, then don't stick with them. Rules like "we only play together" or "always use condoms" or "no anal sex" or "no kissing." Couples develop their own idiosyncratic rules.
- Lying in online pictures. Same as the problem with standard online dating.
- Disagreements on rules. The girl wants one set, the guy wants another.
- The guy tries to steal another guy's girl, typically for one-on-one dating. I have done this before. Sometimes the guy is just fishing and being an a**hole. Sometimes, he senses that he is more masculine or better than the other guy. I only attempt this when I sense strong chemistry with the chick and that I'm better than the other guy.

The main advantage to what I do is volume, sustainability, and of course many people have group sex fantasies; I just happen to live them out.

Doing something like open relationships also takes a lot of self-control and verbal ability... self-control and verbal ability the average person lacks. A guy named Bo Winegard tweeted:

Educated elites who believe that polyamory can be practiced and enjoyed by most of the population remind me of the math professor who believes differential equations are within the grasp of anyone who makes a serious attempt at learning.

There exists compelling research that normative monogamy is beneficial and leads to myriad positive social externalities.

Polyamory is fine as a niche relationship modality, practiced mostly among the extremely WEIRD [Western, educated, industrialized, rich, democratic].

Bo's got a point, particularly regarding people who want real families (see the chapter below on how poly relationships aren't compatible with kids). We're also not willing as a society to have an honest conversation about what's happening below the IQ median. The people driving the conversation at the top really don't have any idea what's happening down there, and choose deliberately not to. They don't really understand what it's like to not have the cognitive capacity to get top-end jobs or have the conversations non-monogamous people need if their relationships are going to survive.

Nash replied:

"Burning Man style: POLYAMORY is more standard than monogamy. Men get the variety they want. They think sharing their women and it's a 'form of love evolution' (they are no longer jealous), but what is happening is it pretty much destroys most of those relationships."

"In 'Burning Man' it's fine to take off your clothes and dance around really sexually. If you were at your grandma's house having dinner (or around children), and you did that, would it 'open everyone's heart?' Or would it create a fiasco? It would create a fiasco."

Nash's replies are notes from David Deida talks. Deida's more right than wrong, because poly/open is a fiasco in all instances except, basically, as casual sex, which is how I do them. Some light swinging can work too, especially in very-long-term relationships, because long-term relationships can get stale and need some more heat. A small number of people can really do open relationships as described. Mostly, "poly" and "open" are about rationalizing casual sex, which is how I use it... because it's a form of normalizing and institutionalizing casual sex for me, I don't get caught up on the terminology.

Kids are challenging enough without all that adult drama. For most people, in effect, poly is a way to f**k around, avoid commitment (avoidant attachment styles are everywhere in open relationships), and enjoy sexual novelty: things I have tended to enjoy. People in "poly" relationships who think they're going to "have a child" together and who are insane enough to execute that plan discover that infants and toddlers are a lot of work, reduce the amount of sex had (for a couple years), and are a lot less "fun" (though often joyful...).

There's a strong tendency to split, to find someone new, unencumbered. Monogamy reduces this problem by the guy making sure the kid is his and the woman making sure the guy isn't out seeding other chicks. Repeat the process of meet-mate-split enough, and you get the epidemic of lonely old people we see in western societies. Even married couples with strong relationships tend to have problems adjusting to kids. The woman's body often goes to hell, for months if not forever... having kids is a great thing, don't get me wrong, but almost no one will do it for kids who aren't theirs. A lot of women also peak in their late 20s and men in their late 30s, so there's that mismatch, which can fuel jealousy. Some people out there appear to experience no or very little jealousy... with the Internet, they can find each other and also proselytize for open relationships, in a way that wasn't possible before the Internet. The Internet lets us learn things and share them widely and also anonymously, and we can learn things we'd never publish in a newspaper or say on TV.

For a guy who wants to be a player, the "open relationships" frame and idea can be a powerful ideology: I don't want to pretend it doesn't have huge costs, though. Many "poly" advocates are simply delusional about its costs, particularly in terms of family and children. Human societies are organized around family and kinship for good reasons, because that's where the genes, love, and mutual interest lie together. As a society, we've spent the last bunch of centuries trying to reorient around strangers and material goods... this has some good things associated with it but it has some costs, too. We've decided to elevate the individual over the family or community... which has some nice features... and some bad ones... we're almost never willing to even state directly that this has happened.

There's an argument kicking around the evolutionary biology communities, that intelligence didn't really evolve to solve problems or be objectively "right," but to form group coalitions and support a given narrative. That may be why "intelligent" people in an IQ sense may be better at self-delusion and maintaining narratives than less intelligent people. We see this especially in places like politics, where most people prefer tribe to knowledge. High-IQ poly people can convince themselves and sometimes others of their narrative, without having the desire to question their own narrative or discover what's "underneath" it. The higher their IQ, the more "reasons" and rationalizations they can come up with. And many of those reasons are real... in specific circumstances.

Poly is probably bad for societies, because it creates male winner-take-most systems. But as people become more individualistic and ever-less connected to family and place, we're seeing the rise of alternate relationships styles. Like old-school Roissy used to say, "enjoy the decline." Or figure out how to make it work. And there are also plenty of chicks out there who aren't participating in the modern mating game... but they're not the ones on the apps, out in bars, etc. They're probably already in a relationship and meet men through family, school, and friends. They're the girls who, if you're not serious about a relationship and family, will disappear right away. Who will stick around if you're not? That's where the game comes from.

Guys with long-term girlfriends

Guys with long-term girlfriends or, worse, wives will sometimes contemplate open relationships, or, worse, have open relationships thrust on them. If the woman broaches the idea of an open relationship, she already has a guy in mind and has either f**ked him or plans to, but the "open" label makes it technically okay. Open-relationship ambush is common and the relationship is probably already dead. She'll get her strange and he will be left hunting online or off. If he has very good game, he might be okay—but if you're living with a woman, you already have f**ked up logistics. You likely can't bring dates back to your apartment or condo. If you do, the girl you're trying to bang will be like, "What's with all the pictures of you with this other woman on the fridge?"

Contrary to what you've ready, most average chicks are not immediately attracted to the idea of being a side-piece. There are some, but they're in the minority. Even chicks having casual sex often like the idea that, if they like the guy, there is a path open to becoming his girlfriend and eventually wife. If you already have a girlfriend or wife, and tell her that, that path isn't open. She can't psychologically justify f**king you by telling herself this could be The One.

There are some girls, a minority of girls, who like being the other woman. They're not impossible to find. But guys with good game start with game that's oriented towards the median girl, then adjust based on the girl's latent promiscuity, the girl's sexual proclivities, the girl's desires, etc. A girl with an apparently slower mating time horizon might still shake out to a lay after three to five dates. Some girls actively want open relationships. Guys ask about fantasies, dreams, experiences, peak experiences, etc. to elicit a girl's values. When I first met Ms. Slav, I was reading a book about psychedelics. That led her to talk about her many drug-related experiences. That's about as clear a signal of being interested in quick sex as there is, short of the girl taking the initiative to unbuckle your belt and fellate you in a bar.

Overall, though, having totally separate open relationships will put the guy in the inferior position, and a woman who proposes a one-sided open relationship has already in effect started another relationship. End it with her and move on. Modern relationships are intrinsically unstable due to an array of conditions beyond the scope of this book, so men must be ready to face the dating market again at any time.

If the guy is contemplating opening the relationship, he needs to be ready for what it means if she says "Sure." If she's imagining that they're both going to have sex separately, with whoever they can find… he is in for a much rougher ride than if he's together. If she wants to go to the sex club with you, and you want to do couple-to-couple swaps, you'll be okay. You'll be on the same team. If she wants to bang Greg from the office tomorrow night, you'll have a problem.

The situations I'm describing, and the problems they entail, are similar to the problems guys have when they're caught cheating. If a guy wants to cheat, it takes a fair amount of time, skill, and effort to make casual sex happen. If a woman wants to cheat, she can ask pretty much any straight man and make it happen. Or spend 15 minutes on Tinder. Women find casual sex very easily. A woman who wants to go cheat and have revenge sex will be able to execute that revenge sex almost instantaneously, whereas guys don't have the same option (except through cash).

This dynamic is part of the reason it's important for a man in a long-term relationship who is interested in open relationships to make sure his woman is on the same page. Otherwise, she may go out and have sex with like 10 guys in the course of a couple weeks or a couple parties, while he's futilely swiping on Tinder. I've seen it happen. I've seen guys cry. I've seen couples fight, when the woman arrives at the party with her boyfriend or husband, then goes off and abandons him in pursuit of d**k. If a woman posts an online dating profile saying she's in a relationship and just looking for fun, she'll have a barrage of d**ks thrust at her. If a guy does the same, nothing.

This scenario also depends on SMV. If you're an attractive guy who hits the gym and has good social skills and you're with a larger chick, you might still be okay because of the SMV mismatch. But then why are you with a fat chick in the first place? If you and your girl have similar SMVs, and you're only offering chicks casual sex and she's only offering guys casual sex, she is going to have an easier time of it.

Non-monogamy comes in a variety of shapes and forms, and it can be used as cover for cheating, or as a form of initiating a breakup without having to be an adult and execute the breakup. Non-monogamy can also be a way for a long-term couple to re-ignite dormant sexual passion. For married men, non-monogamy is more dangerous than it is for women: she can divorce you, marry the next guy, and take half your money and assets

* * *

Despite the caveats above, **non-monogamy saves some relationships**. Will yours be a relationship non-monogamy can save? I don't know. Car wreck stories are more popular than quiet success stories, so you'll tend to hear about people who try a sex club and have their relationship explode, particularly if one or more participants in the relationship goes public with the details. You'll tend not to hear stories about couples who decide to hit the sex club once every month or two and find that it strengthens their relationship and allows them the outlet they need to stay together *and* raise their kids. How many relationships die due to sexual boredom or a desire for sexual novelty?

Men have to create their value. Women have to protect their value. Men create value through a myriad of ways: founding companies, becoming athletes, dominating other men, winning prestige contests, scientific discovery, standup comedy. The number of potential ways to create value is almost limitless. Women, just by being young and hot (or fertile, which is another way of saying "hot"), have intrinsic value to straight men from puberty until the approach of menopause, with younger women being more attractive because they have a larger number of fertile years left. A woman "protects" her value by not indiscriminately sleeping with loads of men. Most women understand this instinctively. That's part of the reason it can be hard to introduce a woman into consensual non-monogamy and keep her going in the scene.

Most women like sex and know a man won't stick around without it. Simultaneously, most women are sensitive to social pressures and to protecting their value. Some women think being in the non-monogamy scene means they don't have to protect their value any more. Usually, such women cannot find primary partners. If a man is with an attractive woman and the woman has sex with lots of other men, she's giving value away—which will draw a lot of potential "customers," who don't have any reciprocal relationship with her.

Other forms of non-monogamy

I've described non-monogamy from the perspective of swingers and polyamorists. There are some other kinds of unusual sex practices you'll discover. Some chicks love BDSM and being tied up but don't like sex very much. For me, BDSM is foreplay designed to get the chick into sub-space, or in the mood for sex, so I'm not very interested in girls who find BDSM as an end state in itself, rather than as a journey into sex. In the rare cases when I've found girls like that, I don't attend much to them; I've only met two hot girls who are like this. One was married and eventually divorced, only for her husband to marry one of their female partners (who liked regular sex).

A few guys are into cuckolding or hotwifing. Cuckolds usually like some element of humiliation; they want to be told that they're inferior to the other guy (often called a "bull"), they want their wives or girlfriends to say the other guy is better. Some want to watch their wives or girlfriends getting f**ked by another guy. "Hotwives" just have sex with other men, usually without their guy in the room, and there isn't an overt humiliation element to the experience. I group these two because they're more similar than not.

The spread of porn seems to have made cuckolding and hotwifing more popular, or at least raised awareness. I don't think it's very productive to seek out couples who are into hotwifing because there simply aren't many, the woman is usually not very hot, and those couples are besieged by guys trying to get free p***y. It's harder to stand out with these couples than it is to stand out on Tinder. Few hot women willing to have casual NSA sex and very large demand for those women means challenge. Many are fascinated by guys with huge d**ks (I'm pretty average). This is a low-percentage play, since demand for free p***y is high while supply is low. Most guys are better off learning daygame than seeking out very improbable bangs from cuckold or hotwife couples.

That said, if I run into this type of couple online or in person, I will sometimes take the easy shot on goal. With this kind of couple, having sex videos or pics on hand and ready to go is key. Because the man is often running the account, he's visually oriented and he'll be interested in the videos. Pre-selection is useful. Most guys don't bang hot chicks, so having a selection of short, anonymized videos demonstrating your sexual prowess is useful. It demonstrates a level of competence that most guys lack. Still, sending videos or pics online to strangers may just be feeding pic collectors.

In addition, most guys who say they're interested in letting their girl be a hotwife, flake. Most guys are also bad at sex, so couples in this scenario will often find a guy who can't get hard, or comes in two minutes and can't get hard again. If they find a guy who isn't incompetent and isn't trying to steal the woman for himself, they may want to keep him around.

The first couple I met who have a strong hotwife dynamic happened with Libido Girl, about halfway through our relationship. The woman in the couple was in her mid-30s but still tight, and the guy was in his early 40s. We met at a party and exchanged numbers at the end of the night. Libido Girl wasn't that into the guy, and the week after we met she was out of town or otherwise unavailable (I don't recall exactly why). The other couple was interested in meeting up anyway, for a drink, and it was a pretty straightforward experience. The guy and I went back to my apartment and took turns banging the woman until the night got late. I kept meeting her, off and on, for the next two years or so, but our relationship petered out because she was rarely my priority. As I got better offers, I was less interested in her. She was also approaching what Red Pill guys call "the Wall," and I was still finding hot chicks in their 20s. I liked her, just not quite enough to keep it going. Her husband didn't seem to care too much about her going out and getting some strange d**k and even seemed to encourage it. I think she got laid more than he did, but I will say that he got a fair amount of sex from various women, usually with his wife's help. I would want a more equitable arrangement than the one he had, but it seemed to work okay for them.

I met another woman online many years ago, and she was part of a couple in which she identified as having a stronger sex drive than her boyfriend, so she would sometimes meet guys on her own. She was on a kinky site, which helps, and we chatted a little online but met in person at a party, where we recognized each other. I was like, "Are you [screen name]?" and she replied yes, then realized who I was, and that gave us an instant rapport (online and offline game are not always as separate as some players would have you believe). I was busy at that party but collected her info, and we met for a drink, came back to mine, had sex, and kept that going for a couple months. Our sexual connection was good but not outstanding, and she was not as available as I would have liked, and I was not as available as she would have liked. But I was better in bed than most guys she found and she was prettier than most girls in her situation, so we made it happen every so often.

* * *

The cuckold/hotwife thing is also rare enough that I hesitated to include this section, but I do so for the sake of completeness and because guys who travel this road may find it. Low-probability outcomes can be achieved. I naturally love the idea of banging another guy's chick with no consequences and no relationship expectation—me, and every other guy.

Couples interested in this seek out strangers, because most guys don't want all their friends to know he's a cuck. Most women don't want their friends to think she's a slut, and thus a threat to the friends's relationships. I personally don't like the word "slut" in most circumstances and prefer the term "sex positive," but the larger culture retains the word and its negative connotations for good reasons. The greatest threat any woman's relationship faces is another woman. So women slut-shame other women in order to guard their male mates. As long as this dynamic persists, we're never going to get ride of the word and the cultural meanings behind it.

"What about STIs?"

People in the sex club community are more fastidious about condom usage than people in the larger community. I've never had a stranger at a sex club attempt to have unprotected sex with me, while I've had numerous girls I've met through normal or online means attempt or encourage it. People in the sex-club scene have a reputation to protect, and they will get a bad rep very quickly if they bring STIs in.

Guys who consistently and correctly use condoms every time don't have STI problems. In addition, it is common in the scene to get quarterly STI tests and share the results with potential partners. People are conscientious about this issue because, if they are not, they will be ostracized. I'm much more worried about sex with randoms from the street or online than I am about people in the scene, due to the reputational effects from giving someone else an STI.

In addition, we already have a vaccine for HPV, and you should get it, if you haven't been vaccinated. Some people worry about herpes, but both prevention and treatment vaccines are close to market (check search engines for details).

There is some risk intrinsic in having lots of sex with lots of people, but I find the reward worth it. People who say, "What about STIs?" usually don't want to go to sex clubs, and that's fine, but just say, "I don't want to go."

People are, or should be, careful about condom usage. I switch condoms anytime I switch partners. I don't think most guys come on their partners's bodies without asking first.

This section is short because STIs are treatable, we're getting better treatments for them every year, and overall they're extremely unlikely to be a problem for people who consistently use condoms correctly.

Sex makes strangers into fast friends

"Which People Would Agree to Have Sex With a Stranger?" is an article from *Psychology Today* that's highly relevant to men in the game. It looks at tests done by aspy psychologists who set out to discover and document the obvious: almost all men say they'll have sex with an attractive female stranger and no women say they'll have sex with an attractive male stranger. That's being asked in daylight, possibly in front of other people, but as players know most chicks take some to evaluate a strange guy. Same day lays from cold opens are possible, they just aren't easy or common. Guys who filter for same day lays are leaving the vast majority of chicks on the sidelines.

There are also gaps between total strangers and strangers

who have some social context. You may notice that colleges and workplaces appear to have more stranger or semi-stranger hookups. That's because familiarity and some shared things in common allow women to feel like the guys they're hooking up with aren't total strangers, and who might suffer from some reputational consequences to bad behavior.

Same thing happens in sex clubs. When a couple first arrives, everyone is a stranger. But most clubs have some regulars and some floaters or orbiters. Floaters and orbiters will also be found on some websites and apps. So even there, the apparent fantasy of "total stranger sex" is rarely indulged. People will often form small friendship groups in which everyone agrees to have sex with the opposite-sex members of the group. On any given night, some number of people in the club are likely already committed to having sex within their groups. Good clubs disallow single men, so at the very least any given man will have one woman who vouches for him. There are **no** unpaid venues where it's common to have stranger sex.

Women who have sex with strangers are more fearless and more open to novelty and new experiences than the women who won't. Women have little to lose by making a man wait a couple of days, and women can assess a man much more accurately over that time: players have figured out that 4 – 10 hours is typically the magic number to go from stranger to sex. Most guys who shoot for very fast sex with strangers will estrange most women. Life does not work like visual porn (male fantasy) or romance novels (female fantasy).

Despite my disdain for social media, I still have a somewhat well-developed account on one or two platforms because girls have reported that that makes me feel more "real" to them. By that, I believe they mean I have real friends, a reputation among those friends, etc., and that makes me feel safe.

For chicks, there is always tension between safety and danger/mystery. Too much safety and a guy is overly weak, boring, and predictable. Too much danger and mystery and the guy is overly risky and might ignore a woman's consent or otherwise injure her without repercussions. Game attempts to teach men to navigate these poles.

For most people, women or men, there's also a point of satiation around sexual urges and novelty. It's not uncommon for a group of three or four couples to form and meet once a week or every two weeks. Who needs the crowds of clubs and the uncertainty of apps? These kinds of arrangements can minimize the shallowness of meeting and learning about new people while also alleviating the boredom that can set in after sleeping with the same person for a long time. You get enough variety to have fun but enough continuity not to feel like you're unmoored.

One word of caution: it's fine to bring your real-life friends with you to sex clubs or parties. But I recommend not swapping with them on the first night, particularly if they are new to the practice, scene, and community. Let them ease into the process. It is a very common pattern for a couple to go to their first sex club, get carried away, do full swap, then regret it the next day, and you don't want to break real friendships or welcome that kind of drama into your life.

Let your friends do full swap with someone else the first time they do it. Let them process their emotions to see how they feel the next day. If she's into you and he's into your date one day, they will be fine a week or two later. No need to raise tension and induce friendship problems where none exist. The full swap can feel very urgent in the moment, but resist indulging until your real-life friends have seen and felt the full experience.

* * *

Hosting your own parties

This is an advanced topic and it won't be relevant to most of you. Many people end up hosting their own parties when their contact list grows faster than the number of dates they can schedule or parties they can attend. I mentioned that it's a fine idea to collect contact info towards the end of the night and meet up with other couples for dates. If you're a social guy and know how to work a room effectively, you can end up with dozens of other couples and girls pretty quickly. Don't know what to do with all those new leads? Got too many people and too little time? Host a little party of your own, either at your place or in a rented hotel room (if the group is small enough).

Hosting your own parties leads to the usual problems of parties, like people flaking, last minute cancellations, uncertainty, etc. But if you can get 12 hot people in a room together you can gain social status in the process plus have a great time. Most guys writing about the game are anti-social introverts, so this may be too much for them. Many of the guys have a systematizing mindset, too, so party planning plays into that.

Some people try to short-circuit the in-person meeting process, and instead try to recruit people from the Internet. This is usually a mistake. The best people have calendars that are too full and aren't likely to commit to events offered by strangers online. Most people do things for others with whom they have an emotional connection. If you've had a positive experience with a girl or couple, they're likely to show up and unlikely to flake out. They worry about their reputation with you, just as you worry about your reputation with them. The tighter your human, emotional bond, the better the party will be. Parties of Internet strangers will fizzle because those people will either not be who they say they are, or they will not show up. The meeting, dating, and vetting process can be slow, but that's because friendship is slow, organic, and person-to-person.

I have heard guys (and only guys) admit they use customer relationship management (CRM) software to track guests, ping leads, etc. If you're in the business world and deal with sales, clients, etc., CRM software will be familiar. Guys with good value, good game, and good environments see their lives overflow with p***y; guys without them always struggle and the need for CRM will be as foreign as life on Mars.

BDSM incorporation and dates

The following is designed for one-on-one dates but can be expanded to two-on-two dates, particularly when you tell one girl to flog or spank another one.

Most guys still don't know and can't do BDSM, but one guy who is working the game says, "I know it sounds a weird request – but how would you stage a sex date with a girl who has complained all her life about sex not being rough enough? I'm planning the date with the MILF for next week."

Not odd/weird… there are lots of things to do… if you have space and money for a spanking bench, that is a nice touch (etsy seems to be the place to buy them, don't know why, but check your local sex shops too). Many apartments/flats are too small for spanking benches. In thinking about BDSM… do the slow/teasing leadup… most girls complain that guys go too fast and are in too much of a hurry… so do the opposite.

If it's one-on-one, start with kissing her, holding her neck, etc. When she is ready, collar her and put wrist and ankle restraints on her. You might use them, you might not. I wouldn't gag her the first time, tempting as it is.

- ◆   Have nipple clamps (key) and a collar.
- ◆   Be ready with a butt plug and lube.
- ◆   Talk dirty, tell her she's a slut, etc.

As you kiss her, strip her. Play with her nipples and see how sensitive they are. Eventually she'll only be wearing her panties (assuming she's wearing any). While she's still standing, bend her over partially, using a gentle but firm hand on her upper back, and begin spanking her. If you've never spanked a woman before, "How to spank a woman" in a search engine will give you good resources. Alternate spanking and caressing. Pay attention to her sounds and body. You may go back and forth with a paddle, or with a flogger.

Engage a leather paddle. Move to a wood one if you think she is not reaching her terminus. If you are swinging a wood paddle like a baseball bat and connecting with her ass... and it is not enough... then she is going into places I (personally) don't want want to go. It's getting too close to something like torture instead of bondage. Some chicks who go for that, but I find it to be a real turnoff when she's into that level of pain/suffering. For newbie chicks, hands and paddles are usually sufficient.

At some point you want to slide your hands in and begin touching her clit. If you've spanked her well and her body responds well, she'll probably be wet. This can go on for as little as four or five minutes or as long as 20 or 30, intermittently, with some gentle caressing in between.

You might move her to the bed at some point, or the bench. Like with sex, it's not a bad idea to move spaces once or twice. Not so much as to break flow, but enough to keep her from getting bored or too acclimated. And go a little more slowly than you think. It's tempting to just ratchet up rapidly. If you sense she's getting bored or restless, ratchet up more quickly.

You can also play with the restraints and with blindfolds. When she's been spanked well, tie her to the bed and try going down on her and you will likely get a great response, for example. At some point just f**k her as you normally would, but incorporate spanking and choking into it. Hold her collar, lightly, perhaps. This can be dangerous because you don't want to hurt her windpipe, so be careful with it.

Like with sex or symphonies, it's good to have some mini crescendos, then back off, then build up again.

Like with business, proper preparation is ideal. For chicks, guys make things "just happen" so that the chick doesn't have to do anything besides pick her outfit and bend over. Chicks live in a world where they just show up… and the guy has done the work… so do the work. Feminism's noise about "equality" is bullshit. Most chicks want an experienced guy to show them the way.

So that's my step-by-step towards a chick who has never had it rough enough. This is a scaleable action plan, because some chicks just want a little light spanking and paddling, which they've never had from their pussy, feminist boyfriends. Some chicks want extreme pain that I don't want to get to. Most chicks won't know where they are until you take them there, and ideally the chick will say "yellow" if you get her to that end state. A good dom is monitoring the chick carefully and backing off when necessary.

I don't think the player who asked really needed the above… it sounds like he'd got it all figured out and was prepared but also ready to change based on the feel of the mood and other contingencies. Being prepared decreases any stress or anxiety in the moment… I have done a little description of prep to friends who say that it sounds like a lot of work. But then I point out that advance work improves the moment because you don't have to worry about where the paddle is, whether the cuffs are available, how to tie her up, how to release her, etc.

Also, you don't have to use the equipment at all, or not all of it, every time. You can just use what feels right and if she's fatigued or you're just done, you can have it and not need it. Like firearms and condoms, better to have it and not need it than need it and not have it.

My sense is that the BDSM market is not tapped properly online, unlike the general market.

Thinking long term

A player I know has discovered a coven of group sex and open relationship people near him. Some of the players are quite wealthy and have oriented their lives around this activity, buying yachts and getting hotel rooms and pimping out their living spaces to make it all happen (the yacht thing isn't necessary, but I guess it's a nice touch if you have the cash... I don't, and I don't really move in those circles... though I know they exist... so don't get caught up in that side alley, whining about income). The player almost can't believe this thing exists, but I can believe it because I have seen versions of it. Non-monogamy and sex clubs become an ecosystem. It's possible to rack up incredible numbers through this, if it is a guy's goal to do so.

Let me try to explain it, from my interactions. I have been at the periphery of this kind of thing but have not been interested in going all the way, into making this the sole and entire focus of my non-work life... a lot of the guys at the top, doing penthouses and boats, are quite a bit older and as a result are not with the chicks who most interest me, but that is not universally true. These guys (and some women)....

* * *

* Go to clubs/events most weekends, or on vacations. There's an international circuit of people doing this.

  * Network with the people they meet. It's not that much different than business networking except it's more emotional and obviously instead of business relationships you are probing, establishing, and maintaining sex relationships. The social aspect of this is important and easy to do poorly. Outsiders think you just show up, bang/mate, separate, like lizards or something. Not really, not if you're doing it well.

  * For guys who want younger/hotter chicks, the trick is finding them. They do show up, by the way. They are just uncommon, obviously.

  * When you have more girls than you can handle (it happens) and are friends with more couples than you can handle, you begin doing parties. Six eight ten twelve people, sometimes more, invite them over and suddenly you are the host and you have the status that comes with being the organizer. Leaders have status… it's polite to thank the host.

  * If you have the money and space to host great parties people will like you better. Chicks are super sensitive to environment and emotional cues. Most guys will happily f**k hot chicks in any available conditions. Dirty sheets, plates in the sink, whatever, guys will happily f**k a hot chick who will bend over there. Chicks are much more attuned to lighting, cleanliness, mood, etc. So if you can just buy the booze and weed, set up the mirrors / beds, get superior lighting (Philips Hue, don't cheap out here if you can avoid it), etc., then people will be more likely to want to attend your things.

  * Really rich guys will buy boats, penthouse apts, penthouse hotel rooms, etc.

It can also take a lot of money to do this. Renting space,

arranging things, etc. Most guys aren't determined to maximize the amount of sex they have, and you can tell as much from their behavior. The chicks who have these fantasies and desire these things will like guys who can activate their fantasies and execute them in a safe and controlled environment. Most chicks also need aftercare, etc. They want to bond, not just be sex toys who are going to be discarded after the event. Many guys wrongly neglect aftercare, cuddling, etc.

Some other things about this big ecosystem…

* Chicks vary in their propensity to engage…. some are super scared, some are pretty eager. Find the eager ones and reassure the scared ones. Obviously a lot of chicks have group sex fantasies, are curious about how other people f**k, etc., but will not explore those without guys to guide them. Be that guy and find other guys who are non-judgmental, etc.

  * If you fully enter and connect to this world you might be astonished by the fact that it is larger than you know… just most people are smart enough not to advertise they're into it… the social judgment is too intense. You'll find business connections in the places you might not expect to find them. Things that start about business often end up being about sex… and things that start about sex often end up being about other things.

  * The people in this world are pretty discriminating, especially when it comes to guys. Many more guys want to get in it than chicks. Even guys who think they want to get in, typically can't handle it. Getting into this world requires people in both sexes who can handle it. Lots of people (guys included) form quick emotional attachments to their sex partners and then want to monopolize those partners… even if they fantasize about this world, it doesn't work. People

who are doing events will monitor newcomers for negative and positive traits and guys (or chicks) who can't handle it will not be invited into the higher tiers of things. Sufficiently badly behaved people will be booted, although this is rare.

In life you are always being judged and always proving yourself.

Real question is…… eventually……. how do you want to live your life?

Most people who learn about this world discover they do not want to spend their lives immersed in it. Just like most guys seem to have about four to five good years in the game… but the people who do keep it up can have experiences few others do.

This no doubt sounds like a lot of work, but… a lot of work compared to what? I know people, even employed people, who spend 20+ hours per week on video games and Instagram, etc. Is this a worse hobby? Think about the things people you know do when they're not working… is this better? Worse? Would you rather be f**king or leveling up your level 29 wizard? Would you rather be getting beers with "friends" from the office or f**king a hot chick?

These things are not very compatible with very young child family life, and a lot of people with kids are too tired to pursue them. As the kids get older it becomes more possible to pursue them but most people in western countries let themselves go, get fat, and get outcomes consistent with their weight, fatness, lifestyle, and sugar intake.

A lot of guys with high numbers also don't have consistently high quality, so there's that.

Some guys spend a lot of time building up their non-monogamy ecosystem and once the machine starts, it purs along. I'm trying to help guys get started and to understand the underlying principles at work. I think the book does that well.

Poly relationships aren't compatible with kids

For most people, certainly: spend enough time in and around sex clubs and non-monogamists and you'll hear advocates say that poly families are "better" for kids because the kids have more adults around who care about their well-being. Realistically, this very rarely works, despite what advocates claim.

For most people, pair-bonding and pair-primacy is necessary for a functional family. Love is pain and all that, so I'm less worried about "someone getting hurt" emotionally from non-monogamy, and more worried about being able to have kids and the family stability that's good for kids. Very few people who really do "poly" seem able to make that work long-term, even among the people who claim that it's better for the kids, etc. Occasionally, male-female-female triads seem to kind of work, if the women are both bisexual and really into each other. In those scenarios, it's possible for the man to work, one woman to work, and the third woman to stay at home with the kids. Realistically, for the overwhelming majority of people in couples (or more than couples), kids change the whole game and introduce a bunch of stressors that didn't exist prior to their existence. Someone who doesn't want kids, can probably make long-term non-monogamy or even polyamory work. Someone who does want kids, or who has kids... it's much harder.

The "swinger" model works much better for most people with kids, or aspirations to have kids. The couple goes out, finds another couple, does a couple-to-couple thing: they have the balanced equations I've been describing, and then everyone goes home and deals with their own spouse's finances, families, emotional needs, mess & clutter, etc.

* * *

The people who are serious about having a family almost always drop out of the open-relationship scene when they're ready to have a family, sometimes for many years... and sometimes forever. Many of the people who think they want to have a family but never quite make it, devote more time to cultivating new partners, new sexual experiences, finding something wrong with their previous partners, become addicted to new relationship energy (NRE), and so on. Most guys in their 20s don't want a family right away, but some guys in their 30s decide to chase the next sexual thrill, instead of focusing on intimacy with one woman. The couples who really make it are the ones who make f**king other people, about being with each other.

Something I have rarely done.

Incompatibility with kids is especially hard on women. A woman dating an attractive guy will see that, as she enters her 30s, he's going to be tempted to chuck her over for a woman in her early to mid 20s. The normal desirability curves still exist. Non-monogamy impedes family formation for most people. Women who are serious about having kids will almost always reject non-monogamy (but they are also probably not the player's primary target).

CHAPTER TWO

Stories

This section is somewhat different: the first section is more abstract, like a textbook explaining a theory. This section consists of stories and discusses a series of lovers who were important in my own life experience and who contributed important understanding to how non-monogamy really works. I don't believe I've ever seen it portrayed accurately in novels, movies, or TV shows, and, as I've mentioned, most books about non-monogamy are very blue pill and are thus missing key aspects of male-female interplay. Most of these stories were written either long after the events in question or while the events were happening, so the perspective changes. I've tried to avoid majors edits to the stories that I wrote contemporaneously.

Metamorphosis: Libido Girl

There are a couple main routes people get into sex parties and non-monogamy. Some, like me, are introduced to it by a lover, in my case "Libido Girl." Others, mostly couples, read about it somewhere, use a search engine to do some research on the possibilities near their city, and start to go. Or they create online accounts to do two-on-two dating. A few learn about the scene through friends and then start to come.

I got into the sex club thing in my late 20s. I'd met Libido Girl through conventional means; she was around my age, and she got into sex clubs because conventional relationships basically didn't work for her because she wanted (maybe still wants) too much sex.

Sounds like a weird, hot problem, right? A normal guy thinks, "Finally, a girl who is unambiguously into sex!" Only if you've never experienced these chicks, who will wear out normal guys. Sometimes these girls get a medical tag like "Persistent genital arousal disorder" (PGAD), or they get labeled as sex addicts. Other women and society can't handle them. Highly-sexed girls disrupt the normal order in a way that makes normal chicks unhappy and even most guys unhappy, because most normal guys want to monopolize a girl, not be exhausted by her until she needs strange d**k and will find it somewhere else.

For some high-desire women, sexual desires mess up their lives. There is a trade-off between "normal" life and your sex life. I personally would prefer a gonzo sex life and worse normal life, but many women feel the tension keenly and it hurts them psychologically and socially. I think the roots of high desire are just biological variation at work. Some are tall, some are short, some are horny, some are less so. Very libidinous girls want serious, hard fucking at least once and preferably twice a day. Often, school is very hard for them, as their desires pull them in one direction while the mass of other girls, who police female sexuality, pulls them in another.

If you're a basic guy you might be thinking, "Great, I'd love it!" You do, in theory, at first. A very high libido woman will often not be able to find men who can keep up with her. So her relationships suffer and maybe her whole life suffers. Word may get around her social circle that she's a "slut" (a word players should not use, as members of the secret society are sparing with that word) and other girls better keep their boyfriends away from her. All very unpleasant things. She may be needy with her monogamous boyfriend, who can't get hard again fast enough.

If these kind of women can separate sex from emotion (not all women can, and that's one reason I'm willing to do more long game than some game guys suggest), they're often well-suited to being escorts or sex workers.

So what's a girl with a super-high libido to do? She can try to find a guy to match her. Most guys, confronted with a wildly sexual woman, will exhaust themselves eventually. Libido Girl had gone through the up-and-down monogamy cycle a bunch of times, until she figured out that she wasn't meant to be monogamous. She found out about consensual non-monogamy and group sex and began going to clubs. I don't remember how she learned. She read something or a guy told her. Quickly she got involved in the scene and then began bringing other guys into it. She'd been going for about two years when I met her.

We started hooking up, and she plied *me* with questions that probed for a sex positive outlook and for how judgmental I am. She was eager to f**k quickly, which told me something, but I got the sense that she'd had a lot of talks with guys about sex and that my answers seemed to fit whatever checklist she was implicitly going down (later, I'd have the same kinds of conversations with many girls).

Within a week or two, Libido Girl asked if I wanted to go to her friends' sex party. That sort of thing wasn't really on my radar then. She was a very popular guest because she was pretty (a low 7 I'd say, but good personality) and feral. Hot, low-drama, high-libido women are always welcomed. In advance, she'd told me that it would be an intense experience. She was right. The party was held in an apartment, and something like 14 – 16 people were there. I met most of them at the beginning. It started off like a regular party… drinks, chitchat, hanging around, flirting. Most women wore more revealing clothes than they typically would. A couple of guys had floggers or paddles hanging off their belts, which is not common at vanilla parties.

After a couple drinks, most of the chicks took off their dresses or fancy clothes. They started kissing each other or their partners. Most parties and club nights have three distinct phases: drinks and chat, metamorphosis, and wild f**king and walking around nude. The better parties close their doors at a predetermined time, which is often the signal for the f**king to start.

At my first party, the metamorphosis was quick. I didn't have a lot of time to register the change. Libido Girl and I were kissing, then she stripped off her own clothes, then she began going down on me on me with the enthusiasm and skill most guys merely dream about. By the time she'd taken me inside her mouth, pretty much everyone started fucking. It was a little bit like visiting a foreign country, because everyone was just doing their thing and so it seemed pretty normal, except for the obvious.

Humans are herd animals, and when everyone around you does one thing, it's just the thing everyone does, and you kind of start to do it too. Libido Girl and I had sex; I couldn't believe all the action going on around me. I understood that some people did such things, and in college I'd had sex in the same room as my roommate and his girlfriend. I was just not fully aware how a lot of chicks will behave, sexually, in groups. Guys who practice the game are often surprised by the first time they nail a chick in a bar's bathroom, and I felt the same sense of unreality, of the curtain parting, of seeing what society hides—and what I am now revealing, in this book.

Libido Girl and I had sex, then Libido Girl had sex with another girl (who she knew well), and I kind of assisted, for lack of a better term. We took a break. Had another drink. Libido Girl basically set me up with this very hot chick who was part of a couple Libido Girl knew already. Libido Girl was smart, so she watched as the other girl and I fucked, then, after I was fully engaged, she had sex with the guy, so that I was too busy to get jealous. I also had no intellectual reason to be angry with her: if I get to f**k a new chick, she gets to f**k a new guy. Reciprocity is the game.

It was an incredible experience. The chick I got set up with was gorgeous, likely hotter than Libido Girl. First introductions to non-monogamy and group sex are important, and Libido Girl managed mine beautifully. Libido Girl and I went to a club a week or two after and I was pretty much hooked. The club wasn't as good as the party, but we got to meet a few cool people. Typical sex club people are in a long-term relationship, often married, and bored with each other: their love has moved from passionate to companionate.

Libido Girl wasn't a real girlfriend, but she was courteous and straightforward about her desires and expectations... like a lot of girls are not. She wasn't ever going to be a real girlfriend in a conventional sense, but eventually I began dating other women and Libido Girl was fine with it. Chicks like Libido Girl terrify normal women, because Libido Girls don't care very much about monogamy. Libido Girl had been the source of a bunch of cheating, from her own admission. She had a fairly regular job, and it didn't seem like sex *totally* ruled her life, but she was not like other chicks and knew it. Girls like her also like online dating, because they can get sex without affecting their social reputations.

I should clarify that I didn't know the details about Libido Girl from the beginning. I learned them in bits and pieces over several months, or more realistically about a year. I wasn't looking for anything serious at the time, having gotten out of a serious thing not too long before. She also figured out that I'm curious, open to different kinds of experience, and non-judgmental. If chicks think a guy won't judge them, they'll say a lot of things they'll otherwise keep quiet. Libido Girl's cornerstone drives and life story came out, just not the way I've presented it. She introduces sexual chaos to a world where the ideological and intellectual default is still monogamy.

I think I got into sex parties as a solution to a problem, or set of problems. The problem is sleeping with lots of different women and doing so somewhat efficiently. Most chicks who start as hookups will eventually ask, "Where is this going?", and that's the beginning of the end. I'm not sure I will ever be fully monogamous again.

Libido Girl was unusual but not unique in her non-monogamy preferences. Girls like her have to find the right guy or guys. Lots of guys like open relationships in theory but don't like them in practice. Libido Girl had to break up with a lot of guys who became emotionally connected to her and wanted her to be monogamous. She'd learned not to accept monogamy, because monogamy would either break her due to her sex drive or she'd cheat on the guy.

The average chick at a sex club is not like Libido Girl, but there are more of her than I first realized. You wouldn't know her proclivities if you met Libido Girl at a meeting or over coffee. She doesn't dress much more provocatively than typical chicks. She just f**ks more, more often, longer, and sooner. If she goes on a first date with someone she likes, she's going to fuck him (or her). She's highly congruent in her psychology, which is not true of all chicks.

Libido Girl and I kept seeing each other casually until she moved for work. She's gotten fat over time, like so many people who love eating sugar.

* * *

Libido Girl also made me fully reconsider my fundamental values. At work, I'm pretty weird by corporate standards. I'm uninterested in things that consume others: houses, cars, TVs, boats, "vacation" houses, most forms of purchasable consumption. Sometimes I just want to ask, "Why do you buy things?" and "Why do you exist?" But that would go from pretty weird to unacceptably bizarre. I love to workout, eat well, read. Inexpensive activities. And of course sex, a hobby that I can't share with others on the job. Too unruly, too dangerous, too disruptive.

Friends who see my place say I "live like a college student," like it's an insult. I'm like, "What's the point of spending all that money on furniture and bullshit?" Seriously, life is about the quality of your relationships and connections to other people. Sex is the ultimate pleasure and also creates relationships. Almost no one cares about your expensive couch or shitty art. Is it clean and functional? Then it's good enough. The vast consumer marketing machine ingests us all. Few can resist. Even I don't resist that well. We can all do better, as human beings.

With Libido Girl, I also learned a lot about the scene. For example, people doing consensual non-monogamy successfully often have quite orderly, regular lives apart from the sex clubs. Most lives can only tolerate so much disorder before they collapse or spiral out of control. To be totally debauched in one area, one must be very stable and responsible in others. Most people in the community are employed and have a secure financial base, too; it's hard to explore alternate relationship styles if you can't pay rent or the mortgage. People on the edge of poverty need to get their financial lives in order before they can be sex party regulars. People on drugs tend to get ejected from the scene because they are unreliable, violate consent, or have other problems.

Libido Girl and I both got what we wanted: the stability of a primary relationship combined with the novelty of sex with new people. We got to live other people's fantasies.

Girl #2

Libido Girl opened me up to consensual non-monogamy and the sex club world. With and without her, I probably had sex with 15 – 20 women in the first year we were together. Conceivably more. Most weekends we'd go to sex clubs or parties. Sometimes we'd date other couples. We found a core group of 10 – 14 girls and couples we'd see regularly; every person has a finite amount of time and energy. It's often hard to find the best chicks online because the best chicks, who know what they want and compromise well, get a boyfriend and disappear. They might appear online after breakups or when they move to a new area, but there is a distinct "market for lemons" problem that has become more severe over time.

Libido Girl and I maxed out our potential social calendar. We went out more than I would naturally. She likely had more action that year than I did, simply because she had greater energy and endurance. Towards the end we drifted more apart, which is a hazard of a lot of sex with a lot of different people. Her job situation was not ideal, and solving it involved her moving. Even before she moved, I began doing some more online dating. This was in late 2000s / early 2010s, when online dating worked better and chicks were not yet glued to their smartphones. I did well at online dating and upped my photography skills considerably and quickly.

Flaking and other bad behavior was common then, as it is now, but I went on dates and figured out quickly that I wanted to sleep with a woman enough to hook her (usually a month of solid, regular sex and dates), then try and get her to go to sex clubs with me. A few of those chicks met Libido Girl, during the overlap. I took one very young, wild, hot, and stupid/flighty girl to a club and she must have fucked half a dozen guys there, of her own volition, then basically ghosted me the next week. Regret on her part, I suspect. Players know that gunning for fast lays with girls can cause the girls to hate themselves and ghost. In the case of this hot, flighty, stupid girl, I wasn't very sad to see her go, because it's important for a pair who go to the sex club to operate as a team; if a girl won't be a member of the team, she is not a good candidate. She will find some other guy and enter his world, and chances are he will either mate guard her successfully, or she will be a true independent operator, happy to attend parties alone.

The next major girl in my life after Libido Girl, let's call her #2, was not as crazily libidinous as Libido Girl, but she liked sex and was pretty uninhibited about it. She was much less forward than Libido Girl. She was feminine and giggly. She had nice energy and was another solid 7 or so. She didn't lead but was happy to follow. She was also very positive, which is good for me, but she did like experimenting with other girls and had a very open mind. I think she was somewhat bored with conventional dating and was 26 when I met her: old enough to have some experience but not yet desperate for kids. As Libido Girl left, Girl #2 moved into her place, and I more or less absorbed her into the friend groups Libido Girl and I had formed. Integration into friend groups is important because it meant continuity among groups over time: I didn't have to re-do all the work that Libido Girl and I had done together. #2 never got into going to the gym with me, but she was young and had good enough genetics for that not to matter at the time.

#2 and I essentially repeated the Libido Girl process: for a year and a couple months we had lots of sex with each other and went to parties and clubs a lot—probably two – three times a month, so a little bit les than Libido Girl, but a decent number. I probably slept with another 15 – 20 girls during that period. My goal was not then and never has been simply increasing the number of chicks I sleep with, so I wasn't trying to maximize that; I was trying to maximize the quality of each experience and each lover.

Guys with low partner counts are endlessly interested in numbers, and guys with high partner counts don't care, and by the time Libido Girl and I were halfway through our partnership I stopped caring about counts, to the extent I ever did. I had figured out how to integrate non-monogamy into my life. Some women ran away from that, but many did not. When a guy truly has "abundance mentality," getting new women can become easy. I learned it then, or fully internalized it.

Not all the women I slept with were incredibly hot, but none were dogs and all met my own internal quality standards. It was common for couples who were unacceptable to hit on #2 (and me), but we were good at politely turning them down.

By now many of the individual parties and club nights have faded into a blur. I know some people keep records of who they did and so on, but I'm not one of them and prefer to exist in the moment.

The most notable thing about #2 was, to me, how easily she slid into the scene. Most of my favorite girls didn't require that much "game" or persuasion. #2 was like that. She was ready to find what I offered her. Things came to end when she wanted to move in with me and get more serious. Which I did not want. At all. Finding the sex-positive and non-monogamous worlds felt like unlocking a superpower.

If I found a girl like #2 today, I might be more susceptible to her arguments and desires. At the time, it felt like the whole world was sexually open to me, in a way that I almost got when I was in college and immediately after, but my skills and mindset hadn't yet come together properly.

Ms. Slav saga

"Ms. Slav" is the name I've given a very young, very libidinous girl I'm still dating as I write this. She is unusual in that she is as horny and sexually free as Libido Girl. She feels alienated from people her own age, which makes sense. Girls her age have no sense of what they truly want sexually; they are driven by what they're fed by the media and teachers; they are scared and inhibited; they are obsessed with shiny things and social media. Ms. Slav is sexually mature and has more sex experience than many people in their mid-20s. She reads a lot of books, thinks a lot, but also has a very high libido. Ms. Slav said something interesting to me: if she is having a lot of sex, she gets hornier, but if she's not, she gets less horny. Other women have made similar comments. It's part of female sexuality being more reactive than proactive, I think. I'm the opposite: when I'm having a lot of sex, it's good (don't get me wrong), but I'm less compelled to seek it out. When I haven't been having much sex, then I get ridiculously horny and want to seek it. Different systems among different sexes.

At the sex club with Ms. Slav, she's hot enough that I have my pick of other partners or couples. Guys who combine some game with non-monogamy see compounding returns. Guys who are known in their area for bringing in hot chicks, in turn get other hot chicks brought to them. I have thought about cooling my involvement in the sex-club scene, but I'm reluctant to throw away the reputation I've built there.

For me, that world is now "easy mode." Ms. Slav and I actually have a girl we're seeing mostly together. Originally the girl had a guy she was bringing into the scene, but the guy didn't want to handle it and she backed off him (this is pretty common). She will find another guy, I'm sure, but for the time being she's been great. Sex has been pretty consistent, in the neighborhood of every other day with either Ms. Slav or The Third (as I'll call her, although I don't know if she'll stick around) or both.

I'm playing the same role for Ms. Slav that Libido Girl played for me. For guys, it is useful to remember that, when it comes to younger hotter chicks, you may be up against guys like me, who can offer chicks crazy shit that they've never attempted. With Ms. Slav, I'm the first group sex; the first time she's used a vibe during sex; the first time she's used a butt plug; the first time she's been to a sex party; and probably a couple of other firsts. I'm not sure she will ever go back to normal sex and dating.

Ms. Slav is more into group sex and non-monogamy than just about anyone else I've met. She's totally sexually uninhibited and, while most people who say they don't experience jealousy are lying, I think she's telling the truth. Most of the truth, that is. She does have a little more jealousy in her than she lets on at first, but I think that's because until me she'd never been exposed to consensual non-monogamy.

There has been too much to recount everything and everyone I've done or we've done. The foursomes have probably been most interesting. She is so young and pretty that she attracts pretty much anyone, online and off, such that I feel like I'm being fed this steady stream of really great food… more than I really want to eat, but as the possibility of it presents itself and I get a whiff, I keep sampling.

It's clear to me why normal women hate women like Libido Girl or Ms. Slav: they are highly disruptive to the social order. They reduce female bargaining power and not a little bit—they reduce it substantially. Because of hate, the

Libido Girls and Ms. Slavs of the world hide who they are. Ms. Slav is too young to have taken on a sex-positive identity, but I believe she is taking one on now, and that identity can help immunize her from female haters. As she surrounds herself with sex-positive sluts, her identity will shift and the hate will mean less to her. This is what normal women hate and fear… another woman who will f**k their boyfriends and not be susceptible to slut-shaming.

Ms. Slav is unusual because she is if anything not discerning enough for my taste. Most chicks don't like most other guys and/or are not really bi. Ms. Slav loves sex, loves it with an array of people, and will have sex with seemingly almost anyone she fancies, and she fancies pretty easily. This makes her a potent weapon but also one with drawbacks. I've had a bunch of sex since taking her to the parties, some with an "8," and it is amazing to watch her merge into the scene. But it is also odd to see someone so uninhibited, to the point where she is less specific than I would like. Usually the opposite happens… I encourage a chick to hook up with other chicks, do her part with other couples I like, etc., but Ms. Slav is not like that.

Ms. Slav has been seeking this kind of sexual permission and opportunity since puberty. She has probably been seeking permission to go wild her entire life and now has it: I wouldn't be surprised to see her become some kind of sex educator or sex missionary more generally. Going to sex parties with Ms. Slav is like playing a video game with God Mode turned on. She's so young and hot that the possibilities are only really limited by the other girl's interests and proclivities.

Ms. Slav reminds me a little of down-to-f**k (DTF) girls I've met online and offline. They like sex and are uninhibited about it and if you match some baseline threshold, she's a "yes-girl." Most girls are not like this, but when a guy finds one he merely has to smoothly escalate. That is another reason normal girls hate the Ms. Slavs of the world: the Ms. Slavs undercut the willingness of guys to invest lots of time and attention in more normal girls. Most normal girls won't have sex within an hour of meeting, but the ones who will, hurt the market positions of the ones who don't.

When I'm dating, I usually probe for interest in drugs and drinking, interest in sharing or hearing sex stories, and reaction to light physical touch. There are no doubt more sophisticated algorithms, but the simple one seems to have worked for me. Ms. Slav has unusual experience in drugs and drinking, although she is not an addict and does fewer drugs than any party girl I've known. But her interest in drugs, drink, and new experiences told me she'd be a fast lay, and she was.

We met a couple off an app, Feeld: the woman is very pretty, more attractive than the guy, and very quiet. We'll call her Peaches (more about her in the next section) At my favorite bar (the staff have asked me about my ways… they have seen a lot) Ms. Slav, myself, and the other guy did most of the talking. Then back to my place, blindfold over the other woman, and less foreplay than I would have thought. Ms. Slav stripped her quickly and began going down on her. I have learned to prolong the foreplay, longer than I think it needs to go on for, and been richly rewarded by that practice. The other woman has sensational breasts and I spent a lot of time on her. Great body overall. Face looks very good in the right circumstances. The guy couldn't get off. I offered some pharma assistance in that regard and he declined. They're not super experienced, not yet, and it's hard to know if they'll get there.

Before them, we had another, bad date, with a couple whose pictures were 10 – 15 years out of date. The guy was a personal trainer of some sort and the woman an administrative assistant. They are the stuff stereotypes against swingers are made of: older, annoying, low culture (but not in a fun way), lacking any semblance of glamour or poise. I noped us out. I like girls who are smart but also sensual. Not a big fan of older, dumb chicks. They were an exception, though. Most people are more or less as they present themselves. Lying in online dating is not a high-quality move, because it wastes a lot of time and doesn't result in much.

I'm starting to understand the whole "mid-life crisis" thing, which I used to think stupid. In most ways my life is really good. Yet I feel somehow hollow, or colorless, a lot of the time, and I'm not sure what to do with that. The old ways seem not to be working for me anymore, but I don't know what the new ways might be. I don't see myself continuing indefinitely down this hedonism path, but I also know too much to approve of some other paths. Some I'm kind of stuck. Many of the earlier life challenges, I have surmounted, or surmounted well enough. What next?

I'm not complaining, mind. If you're my age, have adequate funds for housing and books, and are still railing a Ms. Slav, things cannot be that bad. In the future, however, I might shift away from her and towards someone more substantive.

There are also some very hilarious Red-Pill comments Ms. Slav has made. She's been tooling a try-hard guy for months… he kept trying to get her out last weekend, to a bar he was at, and by one in the morning she finally told him to leave the bar because she wasn't going to meet him. I remarked that I would never put up with that kind of behavior. She said, "I treat different guys differently." He asked if she was home yet… and she said to me, as if she were going to write it in a text, "Baby, I wasn't home. He should know that." He is giving her unearned attention, and while she is enjoying it, it isn't getting him anywhere. He texted her that he would rather be out with her than anyone else in the world. This to a young girl he barely knows. Folly. I made those mistakes... in high school and college... not for a long time. If anything I err towards not giving enough attention and not doing enough comfort.

Ms. Slav has required very little training, though. With her... I think I can keep up, but I don't think I want to keep up. Seems like a minor distinction, but I wonder if she's my last ultra-high-energy girl. One down side of guys dating chicks half their age is that those chicks can be much higher energy.

New girl peaches

I said, "I've been in a sex whirlwind," and that is still true. Ms. Slav and I met this couple (pseudo-couple, I now know) off an app, went out, had a good time getting drinks, and brought them back for sex. It was good, very good for me. But as we were moving to it, Peaches dropped that she is... married. Not to the guy she's with. Interesting. I asked if he's a low-sex-drive guy and she confirms, or claims, that he is.

I don't get why a girl like Peaches would get with a low-sex-drive guy. Peaches comes from a somewhat religious family, so maybe she has Christian baggage impeding her. Whatever the case, she has been on birth control since she was a teenager (originally not primarily for contraceptive purposes) and hormonal birth control has not harmed her sex drive a whit.

Both the guy and Peaches are in their 20s, the girl finishing up grad school and no doubt figuring out what to do next. A side thing, a rant really, on grad school: do not go to grad school and then think you're going to get a professor job. This is false for the vast majority of graduate students. The overwhelming majority of people I know who do graduate school get slower and slower and slower as they move through and realize there is no good job for them at the end. I know guys (and some chicks) who are intellectually smarter than I am, spend 6+ years in school, then get post-doc jobs for $50K a year… less than I was making at 24.

For an intellectually inclined guy, it is okay, straight out of school, to do a two-year master degree, then get out. With a master degree, a guy can do some teaching if he wants and if he can make it work around his real job. Teaching can also be a powerful ecosystem tool for getting chicks, but doing graduate school and thinking, "I can get chicks this way" is an awful way to think, but I do believe I have seen it. A guy is better off with a real job and learning game.

Modern academia, like marriage, is a trap. "Smart" guys who are praised by their college instructors may think academia is a good idea. It is not and it will frequently f**k up your life. As it has for Peaches. She is almost certainly making less money than she would have with an undergraduate nursing degree. She is smart and motivated enough to get through graduate school, and that means she could be a nurse practitioner by now and making $90k+ per year. Instead, she makes far less money than that and works to advance someone else's career.

Still has incredible tits, though. Nice body overall. Perfectly shaped and proportioned T & A. Can't figure out why she would marry a guy who is borderline asexual. Ms. Slav has shared some rides with Peaches, and Peaches is pretty dissatisfied with her marriage (can't say I blame her, if what she says is mostly true). Some reasonable number of women doing group sex and open relationships are freshly divorced or out of long-term relationships and ready to party. This one isn't divorced yet, but late 20s and high sex drive + asexual husband equals divorce. The husband knows about her sex life. I don't get him.

I like Peaches's face a lot because I like her as a whole package, but she's got a pretty normal, girl-next-door face. I think she's getting pretty intensely into me. We have great sex chemistry. I'm going to try to break her off from her other guy... I'm better than him in bed, despite being something like 15 years older, and I can see Peaches looking at me and... thinking. Thinking about what she's going to do next. I've been around a lot of girls who are thinking about the branch swing. There is a lot of "money doesn't matter in game" and "don't be a provider" comments in the game and Red Pill community. The first one is untrue or slightly true: money isn't very important in the very short term, but as soon as you get into a regular thing with a chick, it starts to matter if you have none of it. Chicks prefer guys with their shit together, if possible, just like guys prefer younger-hotter, if possible.

It is true that average, game-unaware guys overestimate the importance of money and default towards presenting themselves as providers, both being mistakes. But I see game guys default too far in the other direction. In this foursome, I end up controlling a lot of the narrative and logistics because I have the money and space to pull them off.

So... does money matter? Yes and no. All else being equal, more is better. The older a guy gets, the more true this is. I've seen it go every which way in my life. I've seen chicks leave pretty well-off guys who bore the chick. She goes off with some couch-surfing guitarist. I've seen chicks leave cool artsy alternative guys when the chicks want someone stable and responsible. There is no magic "right" answer because the right answer varies by the chick and how long you're going to be with her. The longer you're with her, the more the money matters, but many guys mistakenly think money is everything, when it's not. Most normal chicks prefer a fun, interesting, lively guy who makes less over a dour, tedious, workaholic who earns more. Even for Peaches, I see her interest in me. Helps that I've banged her unbelievably hard and thoroughly.

A while ago, I was seeing this girl, I think I met her online (so quite a while ago). In her clothes and especially her tight wrap dresses, a good choice on her, she looked delicious. Completely fecund. Curvy in all the right places. I've been with girls like that, and when they're young, they're fantastic. Eventually got her naked and everything flopped out and down. Like unwrapping an anticipated Christmas present that turns out to be old socks.

I've had the opposite happen too. Peaches is the opposite. She looks good but not stunning off the bat. Most guys would probably give her a very high 6 or low 7. Sometimes you'll see some chick you think is okay, she doesn't wear very flattering clothes, or she does but you don't quite know what you're going to get, and you take it all off and everything is perky, smooth, beautifully flush, and you bump her up a couple notches. You just don't know till you close her.

Peaches is more the latter. Looks okay clothed and better nude. I have unusual experience in comparing chicks clothed to chicks nude, due to group sex.

I believe Peaches found this guy, Other Guy, started an affair with him (or talked to her husband first about her sexual needs not being met? I don't know the story yet) and he's sort of "the first person available." Now she's seeing a guy like me, a better choice in almost every way, and I think she is going to wind up with someone else. Such is the danger of non-monogamy for guys who do not measure up, as I think this guy does not.

I was walking out with him one night and mentioned my plans to hit the gym the next day. He was like, "Yeah, I should really get in that." I told him the truth, that I love it, and that I love straining against the iron. I didn't love it at first, but the love grew over time, especially reading some inspirational literature from Arnold, and from other guys who live life in the Temple of Iron. I'm not one of them... I'm not huge or jacked... but I do love chasing the challenge, the feeling of blood rushing into the muscles. A guy who does non-monogamy is going to run into guys who are serious about lifting and diet. That is a danger for the average guy, who is serious about neither, and whose lack of seriousness shows.

I could be wrong. I could try to pull Peaches for one-on-one and fail. It has happened before. But the signs are there. When I first wrote this section, I planned to try to get Peaches out the next weekend, and it worked. I sound awfully arrogant in this section. I'm trying to be honest, though. I have met guys who are better looking and wealthier than me. This one... just isn't one. Sorry, Other Guy. He's also a little too PC for me. A little too SJW. Which is fine... I don't dispute these things all that much in real life. I lead by example, not by derailing good flirting with political talk. But it, his PC-ness, makes me think a little less of him as a man, and it probably also makes normal women just a little bit drier towards him. To normal women, the PC / SJW thing is fine among low-status, non-sexual "allies," but not so good in guys they actually consider f**king. I just don't see those PC / SJW guys getting as much. PC / SJW talk is a demonstration of lower value to women, even women who might agree intellectually.

Being with Ms. Slav has been a wild f**king ride, and it continues to be one. I don't know how long I can do it, though. She parties harder than me. She is amazing in some ways, too much in others. I'm happy to have found her, but I also feel like she is going to be, if not the last, then one of the last girls I do the full, complete, crazy non-monogamy party thing with. The desire is not there as it used to be. But I'm also happy I brought Ms. Slav in. She would have found it eventually, and she is too highly sexed to be suitable for conventional relationships.

She is also less discriminating than most girls and less discriminating than me; girls vary in their personalities, and, in her case, she seems to either be "pansexual" (genuinely is interested in a person's mind) or, more likely, she loves to fuck and is less hypergamous than some girls are. Usually I control the whole flow from meeting to sex. Ms. Slav is happy to have a LOT of sex in one night, and she has it with people she shouldn't, in my view. Not that the sex is wrong, but both the guy and the girl in a couple need to bring value to the table. If they do not, she should not be with them, in my view. I have very much internalized the "exchange of value" paradigm that I have written about. Ms. Slav, when she gets turned on, is not as devoted to that paradigm. Very, very unusual.

She says that she has never done online dating, which is surprising to me. It may be that she is willing to f**k whatever guy happens to be in her orbit, so she doesn't need it.

With Ms. Slav, I think I have changed her entire life trajectory. Her inclinations were already there, but I have opened a door for her. Given her a Red Pill (though not that Red Pill).

I find myself feeling oddly lonely at times, as I have not, usually, in the past. Sometimes in the middle of group sex I feel totally alone. I do not know what that means. Something in my psychology is changing.

Ms. Slav is so young that she is the object of virtually every man's desire. It has been some time since I've been in the scene with a girl quite as stunning as her, and the sheer ease of being in the scene with her keeps me attached to it. Almost any girl becomes available. There is an addictive quality to having that be true. Not having to work hard for high-quality tail is extremely appealing. It's what drives men to the heights of artistic achievement. I don't want to overstate it, as I don't have a free buffet of 8+ chicks, as high-end actors and musicians do. But I have had and do right now have access to chicks most guys would be quite pleased to nail even after a lot of work. Ms. Slav has beauty and I have reasonable game + connections + logistics. Part of me wants to scale back, as you can tell from reading this. Part of me, however, has stumbled into this amazing situation.

Ms. Slav, like a lot of hot girls, doesn't understand that sex isn't just available "on demand" for guys. If she wants sex, she just gets it. Pretty much every straight man she's ever met wants to have sex with her. For 98% of guys, it ain't like that. But for guys, it's often useful to act like it's like that. As I do with Ms. Slav.

I think back now to opening Ms. Slav. Every time a guy opens... he doesn't know what's going to happen. He's making things happen. Women very rarely make things happen. Things happen to women. Even Ms. Slav, who is more forward than most women, primarily reacts.

As of this writing, both Ms. Slav and Peaches are still in play. I don't know what will happen with either. But Peaches came directly out of my relationship with Ms. Slav, which shows how one girl can be used to leverage another.

About a week after I wrote the section immediately above, I met one-on-one for tea, where I showed her my clean STI test results (she knew immediately why), and then back to my place. Very long, very intense foreplay session, complete with a paddle, blindfold, nipple clamps, and an eventual butt plug, as she'd mentioned an interest in double penetration but had never used a butt plug during sex. Now she has.

And it was great. The kind of sex everyone craves and we sometimes don't get. It's smart to wrap it up. But it's so much better bare. We hit a lot of positions, with me directing the show the whole time and her loving it.

I think most guys would rate Ms. Slav as being hotter. She is at the very least 10 years younger. Yet with Peaches, it was just intense. Extremely intense. We may just have a subconscious, sub-linguistic compatibility that Ms. Slav, for all her virtues, does not have with me.

After, I was exhausted and took a brief nap with her in my arms. Then Peaches opened up more about her husband and what a good man he is. This wasn't fun to hear about, but I've had so many of those, "Oh, this is the side of women that women don't emphasize" talks that they don't elicit an emotional response from me anymore. They are just part of the game. The gap between the private narrative and public one is so wide. I think that's why I like game blogs and have for a long time. I resisted starting one because I wasn't sure I had enough material and because I knew that, if I started writing it, it would consume too much of my life. I was right on that second point.

With Peaches, I still can't figure out why she married her husband. She might not be able to figure it out, either. Or it might be that chicks are random, a theme I discuss often. In this post, among many others. But I wasn't highly analytical yesterday after sex. I also don't care very much about what led Peaches into her baffling marriage. I am 85% certain she is going to divorce, sooner or later.

That is what people call afternoon delight.

So delightful that I was still tired when I woke up the next morning. I felt like wasn't on my best game at work. Sometimes after f**king, my mind is so crystal clear that I get everything done and throw off a ton of new ideas. Sometimes I'm still in that half-dream state and need to pull myself into the now.

When Peaches left she looked at me and said, "I needed that." Probably my second-favorite thing to hear from a woman, right after, "Come inside me."

Bike girl doesn't know who she is anymore

I originally met Bike Girl while riding: I came to a tricky section, and a girl was slowing down in front of me. I told her to take lead, and she told me to, so I did. When we passed the tricky section I slowed down and said that I was glad we'd gotten through there. She agreed and I asked where she's going. She said yoga (a good sign) and I told I'd been trying it as a supplement to weightlifting. A little too gay and friendly, maybe, but it popped out. We talked about yoga and I told her to wait at the next light, because I want to get her number.

At the light I pulled out my phone and gave it to her and said that life is like waiting at the light: if you don't act quickly the opportunity goes away.

A pretty basic interaction overall, but her energy was high. I've promised myself that I'm going to stop hitting on women and dating for a while in order to recover myself, but that morning I slipped into old habits. When you've conditioned yourself to flirt as long as I have, you get used to acting in the moment. She gave me the phone back and I said I looked forward to seeing her and gave her hand a little squeeze. That surprised her. Not sure if it's in a good or bad way.

The first date with Bike Girl went very simply and very well. Before the date I did (or attempted) four warmup sets and got harsh blowouts from all of them. A very strange run, but then Bike Girl herself liked me a lot from the get go. She is more

141

shy and introspective than she first seemed, when I think the riding had raised her spirits and also mine. But so far everything seems to be going well. She is also too young to make long long-term work. But I am enjoying the moment and am not going to complain when the right girl at the right time falls into the lap.

Our dating proceeded normally, and I invited her to the first sex party after a month or two of dating. Like most chicks, she was apprehensive at first, but I soothed her and eventually she followed my lead to some fun events. After we'd been going to parties and couples dates for a while, Bike Girl told me, "I don't know who I am anymore," and she was referencing sex clubs and group sex dates. I brought her into the scene through normal means, by dating and having sex, and, about a month in, I invited her to a party some friends were hosting, and she agreed to come.

But I didn't handle her as well as I could have, I think because I've been through this before and I couldn't get up the emotional affect necessary to deal with it properly. Instead I was half engaged during the conversation and that confused her. She seems worried about losing me.

I reassured her that she is a good girl and that I'm watching out for her and that she doesn't have to do anything she doesn't want to do. I think she fears losing me to other women at sex parties. For kind of good reasons. Sex with a new person is very intense and humans, especially women, are primed to pair bond with guys they have sex with. I don't know how to say this without being arrogant, but I combine looks/masculinity/presence and career/money/earning effectively, or more effectively than most guys. Most guys do the one or the other. Realistically, most guys do neither, but most attractive, dominant guys have weak careers and most strong career guys are fat and repulsive. They look like they've spent their life on their careers.

Bike Girl is having both an identity and relationship crisis (or doubts) at once. We've been talking explicitly about open relationships and how to live non-monogamously, and for her I think it's a lot to take in. For most girls it is. Some chicks have been searching for this kind of thing for their entire lives and take right to it, but they're in the minority.

It takes a lot of re-programming to get an average woman into a non-monogamous mindset. There are non-average women who like sex enough, or who have sufficiently damaged emotions, to jump right in. They're the exception. It may also depend on who has greater investment in the relationship. Since I'm almost always less invested than the woman, the woman is more worried about losing me. But with non-monogamy, she can lose me two ways: she can lose me by agreeing (and thus seeing me have sex with other women) but she can also lose me by not agreeing (because she's not doing what all those other dirty chicks will do).

She's caught, psychologically, in other words, and one night I saw Bike Girl thrashing in this trap. This contradiction. To her it's all new. But to me it's not. I've been in it for long enough to see the problems. Because of my relative experience, I've held back more, and let her take a lot of the first steps with others, and worked to let her get comfortable. For example, it's common for a person (guy, realistically) with a new partner to let her be the focus of the other couple, and for the person (guy) not to have sex with the other woman the first time, in order to let the partner acclimate.

I've done some of that. Her uncertainty was also a reaction to a couple we saw on New Years Eve: the woman is incredibly beautiful, and she makes Bike Girl nervous. Bike Girl is in the same league but the blonde is at least a solid point higher. The blonde's guy seems to have his virtues but I think I'm a bit better and kinkier in bed than he is. I think Bike Girl is worried about the heat between the blonde and me, which is not quite matched by what is between her and the other guy.

This is speculation and I don't know for sure, but it does match experience and what I know of female psychology, as well as Bike Girl's personality. Bike Girl has been with me long enough to be past the casual stage, so she wants to figure out if she's going to be with me and non-monogamous over the long term, or with me and make me monogamous, or if she should get rid of me and protect herself emotionally or psychologically. I respect that last choice, too. It may be the rational one for her.

When I wrote this piece, didn't know where things would go with Bike Girl. I think she knows or suspects that, on some nights when I've not been with her, I've been with other women. Not a lot of nights, but definitely a few. I frankly don't have the time or sexual energy to have boundless relationships anymore. Sex every other day is now plenty for me (in college I'd prefer twice a day).

I don't explicitly reveal that I've seen other women to Bike Girl: I don't rub her face in it, and I'm not trying to be mean to her, but I feel the need and have the means to gratify the desire. I've also done less of this simply because she is very good at meeting my sexual needs, and I think she knows that the better she is about that, the better things will be between us. But she's also figuring out that on a lot of weekends I'd rather do sex parties, or a specific number of other things, than I would like to do her dumb chick activities. I tell her to do those alone and she is torn: she wants to be with me on the one hand but knows my independent nature on the other. In some ways I'm very patterned, very mechanical, choosing a small number of activities very specifically. Some chicks get bored with my way of being. They want me to go to a concert… I haven't been to a concert since I was a teenager. They don't like that I don't care about their friend's birthday or about seeing that movie or doing stuff for the Instagram pic.

I think Bike Girl also isn't that used to guys with options. I get the sense she's used to "dating down." I don't know why, because she has a great body, but I think her exes have either been very short FWBs or guys who are more into her than she was into them. So now she's in a reversed situation and it disorients her.

Oh yeah, and somewhere in the midst of it I told her that I love her, which I probably shouldn't have done either. Oops. I have a thing about telling chicks I love them… usually during sex… then never mentioning it again. Probably bad game and bad for the chick's emotional health. But I did it. Can't take it back now.

Bike Girl understands a lot without being able to articulate what she understands. Like I think she understands that a person who is really serious about fitness and diet is also serious about sex. Why is a man so diligent about the gym that he won't be thrown off by female needs? Because he's serious about finding another woman if the current one doesn't work out. Other women have also seen my obsessions with swimming, working out, and not eating sugar as a threat to them. And they're a little right about that.

Sometimes a week or two off restores me to equilibrium. For the player, the first problems are around getting sex with enough girls. Over time, the problems become about relationships, not sex. Because girls can get sex whenever they want, merely having it is not the problem. Getting a high-status guy to commit is the problem.

When I was being Bike Girl, I didn't know if she would re-mold her personality, break, or suffer. They all seemed possible. But with me, she came to accept this as her new normal. Re-molding a personality is very hard and I've been through it multiple times. Being outside the mainstream and outside typical cultural expectations has its costs.

Bike girl was good in many ways, but I like to say, "A kid can get away with having potential. An adult must convert potential into achievement." Bike Girl has potential that she was not converting into achievement. She was fun in bed, with a personality that worked with mine, in that stage of our relationship. But she eventually wanted to move in with me (after not even dating for a year), and when I said no, that brought our relationship to a close. She tried to girl-close me faster than she should have.

I likely would have broken up with her eventually, anyway. For a short-term relationship, most men don't care about a woman's work life or earning potential. For a long-term relationship, this becomes much more important, because smart, balanced, capable women get their work lives sorted out. A woman over age 25 who is still dithering about work is communicating that she is likely not a good, capable, long-term partner. When I evaluate a woman for a potential long-term match, two jobs in particular stand out as being attractive: "teacher" and "nurse." Both are common, good, steady jobs that don't require a lot of career arc and consistency. Both jobs allow the woman to take time off to have kids, then re-enter the workforce if she wants to.

Addendum: Bike Girl and I ended our thing after about seven months, when she wanted to move in with me because her lease was expiring. I don't like the idea of cohabitating with women at all, and I really don't like the idea of allowing a somewhat flakey, somewhat directionless woman to move in with me.

Discretion and the secret society

* * *

Years ago, a lover learned about a mutual acquittance I'd fucked before her. My then-lover was shocked and wanted to know why I hadn't told her. My answer: I don't gossip about sex and respect my lovers' confidentiality. Alternately, you could say, "Would you be happy for me to talk with other girls about what we do together?" That kind of answer is terrible to use with most women, because it's too logical, so I added that I will also respect her confidentiality. I'll apply the same standards to all my lovers. Chicks want you to break the rules for them, of course, but not for other people. Few chicks understand consistency.

I told her to think about what will happen in the future, when she finds a provider guy to have kids with. Does she want me running around, blabbing to whoever, that we had sex?

She weakly argued that she wouldn't care. I told her that both her and I know that's not true.

It's good practice not to tell current lovers the real, full names of past lovers. Let them find out on their own, if at all. If a girl gets mad about your past, promise them discretion in the future. Live that way and you will reduce problems for yourself.

The major exception to this rule is women who are deeply and congruently in the sex party scene. They are typically not as sensitive and will often be open to threesomes and group sex. For normal girls, however, reputation is paramount and guys who can shut the fuck up will help preserve their reputations. Let girls talk about the guys they've fucked.

As a guy, you also don't need to brag about your past conquests to women. Women will be able to tell if you're sexually experienced just from how you are.

Fiona

* * *

I met this girl Fiona online; she was a fairly typical 7 in her 20s, dark hair, slender body, middle height: the kind of girl most guys would be happy to f**k but not special otherwise. She'd finally gotten out of her long-term college relationship, explaining that her and her ex-boyfriend had "grown apart" or some such female nonsense that means, "I want to have casual sex and I was bored with him." Nothing wrong with that, I should add, but it's useful to translate euphemism into reality. I wonder if Fiona cheated on the guy before the breakup. She also should have considered non-monogamy.

Regardless, she seemed up for it on the first date, and I liked the sex so we began seeing each other every other day or so. After a month I proposed taking her to a sex club for the first time, both for my own interests and because she seemed experimental and ready to party. I'd talked to another couple who I knew were going to be there… meeting another couple in a sex club, or for drinks before the club, can be a less intimidating experience for new girls.

At first Fiona was a hard no. She also wanted to go to a concert that night, as she was far more into music than me. I'd gone to a few shows to indulge her, and she'd been to a few of the nerdy events that I like to indulge me, but it was clear already that our default, non-sexual modes of spending time together were incompatible. I'm also leery of girls who love music, because that means they want to f**k musicians and DJs. Since I am neither, I know what will happen. Music and concerts highjack the brain, putting people into a sexualized frame of mind.

Fiona did have many questions about sex clubs and parties, which I answered, giving some of the material you've read in this book, albeit not in this order and without evolutionary biology or game attached. I emphasized that this experience was like a magic mushroom, an alternate reality ride for us, and that it is about us having an ecstatic experience together. Fiona claimed to never have had sex in the same room as another person, even in college, and that she'd never done more than briefly kiss another girl. She said that she only likes men, which I believe, based on later evidence. I told her that she would be the center of attention and that I'd paddle her in front of the entire room, as she was extremely responsive to BDSM and me spanking her was a standard part of foreplay.

She also had some of the spoiled princess only-child effect. Not too much of it, but enough to be noticeable. Most girls like submitting to a romantic partner, but she seemed highly perturbed when she didn't get her own way.

After a couple days and lots of talking I convinced her. As I mentioned, I pitched the event as being part of us getting closer, and I told her that my two friends would come over to pre-game, or we would meet them. Fiona was put out by the fact that I'd had sex with the other woman, but I told Fiona, fairly truthfully, that I had once, in the context of group events. I explained that the other woman was in a committed relationship with her partner and I didn't want to interfere with their relationship, just as they wouldn't want to interfere with our relationship. We went through the "best experiences" and "life highlights" talk, and Fiona's were pretty lame. I guessed that she'd not had really good sex before, and she denied it, saying that she had had great sex with her ex in the first year they were dating.

"What about the other four years?"

"It was okay."

So she spent a bunch of her prime years having sub-par sex…. and for what? Nothing, from what I could see. Many couples see sexual tension grow slack over time and that sex clubs can be a way of renewing good sexual tension and helping a couple stay close. She agreed to go, and we didn't go to the concert that night.

I told my two friends about Fiona, about how she was new and extremely apprehensive, like someone giving up college to start a company instead. Both my friends were familiar with the process of breaking in new girls, and we planned to let her be the focus of attention, just as Libido Girl made me the center of attention when I began going with her. They both came over for the pre-game and were very solicitous, asking Fiona questions and making her feel at ease.

Unfortunately, the club that night was very bad. The only attractive people there were the two of us and my two friends. Fiona and my female friend danced quite a bit, and the other girl showed Fiona some of the toys we'd brought. We put on a good show, and the three of us did spend serious time paddling and spanking Fiona, who had her first orgasm while the three of us were clothed. When we moved to the primary play space, other couples kept trying to join us and I had to keep telling them, "no." A good show for a bad audience. A great comedian in New York City will be wasted on a crowd of rural Mormons from Utah.

You never know which nights will turn out to be golden and which will turn out to be filled with older fatties. If Fiona had been more experienced, I think the four of us would've left and made our own party. But I wanted to fulfill my promise of making her the center of the show. The other girl went down on Fiona (even very straight girls will usually accept oral sex from other girls, as long as none is expected in return) and the other guy had sex with Fiona, as did I. So that went well. The next morning I had to deal with Fiona's concern that she was now just "a dirty slut," "a whore," etc., and I attempted to steer her into the frame that humans like sex, sex is good, and she shouldn't be ashamed of her sexual desires or the kinds of sex she's having. Whether by reason of internal inclination or cultural upbringing, I could never fully sway her into my sex-positive frame.

Fiona was bad at reciprocation and had intense jealousy, and she wasn't interested in FMF threesomes. We did have one, and it was fine, except for Fiona crying after. She did like the chance to have sex with other men but did not fundamentally want me to have the chance to have sex with other women. Her forebrain understood that equality in opportunity is important but her hindbrain wouldn't let go. Throughout our mini-relationship, she tried to make me more monogamous and more invested in her, while I tried to make her less monogamous and more invested in group sex. There is a saying, "You can't make a hoe a housewife" (which doesn't seem to be true, as I have seen exactly that happen), but it's also sometimes not possible to "Make a housewife a hoe," as I was attempting to do.

After a few months, Fiona began complaining that I gave other girls more of my attention than I gave her, that I didn't really care about her, that I was just using her for sex, etc. Players may interpret these as female shit tests, but in this context they were actually comfort tests: she was concerned that I would break, or was breaking, her heart. Early on, I could dismiss them with humor ("Really? I'm worried that you are just using me for sex, just like the last five girls I dated"), but these kinds of complaints became more intense as time went on. I couldn't re-frame Fiona into becoming a sex-positive person. If I met someone like her today, I might consider her as a long-term relationship and as someone to have a kid with. When I knew Fiona, however, I was not interested in that route.

She never really got fully into the scene. Fiona is a girl who was willing to indulge group sex for my sake, and someone who merely indulges will grow less willing to indulge as the relationship becomes firm. Amusingly, she had a cute friend who was probably a high 6: bangable but nothing special, and the high 6 had heard all about our adventures. After Fiona and I broke up, this girl wanted to try going with me, so I took her and banged her for about a month, with my interest declining each time we had sex.

The girl knew it and tried to compensate with ever greater skill and enthusiasm in bed, along with promises of fidelity to me and threesomes to come. The more she craved and sought me, the more I pulled back, and the more she pushed forward. The dynamics reminded me of being in high school and early college, when I had inadvertently strong game with girls I was marginally interested in, but I turned into a b***h around the hot girls I really liked.

With Fiona's friend, it was genuinely easy to be uninterested because being hot/cold wasn't feigned. She was willing to come over, get bent over, and I was okay with that because she was zero work. Fiona naturally got wind of this and sent me a bunch of furious texts. I just told her that she'd broken up with me, so I didn't see the big deal, which was true. We all know, intellectually, that when we break up with someone, that someone is likely to go find someone else to f**k. Fiona had even kept banging my threesome buddy, who I mentioned earlier in this book, and I was fine with that because I had no claim on her and he'd also been good at passing me girls. Him and I had an understanding and were not trying to get one over each other.

Fiona is a good example of the common tendency towards hypocrisy among humans. She verbally and consciously recognized her own hypocrisy, in that she was happy to have sex with other men while she became unhappy with me having sex with other women, but recognition was driven by her intellect while her feelings drove her behavior. I still enjoyed my time with her and am glad were able to do many of the things we did, but we were never in harmony. Her intellect couldn't adequately change her feelings for us to work.

When we broke up, I kept encountering her profile online, as I immediately started doing conventional online dating again, and she did the same. Online dating seems to make real relationships harder to sustain.

Michelle says "no"

I'm pretty sure I met "Michelle" online and we'd been dating consistently and casually for about a month, or maybe a little more, when I suggested we try going to the local sex club (though I didn't phrase it like that; I usually ask if she's up for an adventure, then ask her if she's ever thought about having sex in front of other people, then the questions branch from there. Most girls have this fantasy. I eventually tell her I want to go, then field her questions). She was exceptional because she didn't reply immediately to the sex club part. Then she said no and something like, "You are too experimental for me."

It's one of my favorite rejections, ever. After that, I never saw Michelle again. I probably tried to keep banging her by inviting her out over text, but, assuming I did, she didn't bite.

In retrospect, I think Michelle was looking at me as a family-oriented guy who she might have kids with, and while she was imagining a house in the burbs with a salaryman, I walked into that imagined white kitchen and took a huge dump all over the floating cutting-board in the center of the room in her fantasy. I also diagnose her as looking for a family guy and reading me as a family guy, only to realize when I asked her about going to a sex club that I'm not a family guy and I'm not going to be *her* family guy. She got the feedback she needed and left. Many players hear the "Let's just be friends" talk or a firm "no" and never contact the girl again: there is no reason to if she's uninterested in sex.

Michelle was a slower close for me. It's pretty rare for me to get to the end of a third date without a bang, and I was heading that way with her on the third date because she verbalized to me that she wanted to "take it slow." But I had realized a favorite, magic phrase with chicks who are husband-hunting: "Sexual compatibility is extremely important to me." Sometimes followed-up by, "If we don't have sexual compatibility, nothing else is going to matter." Most American girls in big cities will f**k on first or second dates, and waiting past the third date can be a demonstration of lower value (DLV). I'm not completely against waiting four or five dates for a girl who seems on but pulls back; some girls have an internal three-date rule, but she might be on her period during the third date.

With Michelle, I'll say that true husband-hunters are in the minority, but they are out there, particularly in the late 20s and early 30s. Usually they will make an "exception" for fun-loving bad boys, but not always. Sometimes I anger these women because I can read as husband material to a motivated woman, and when she discovers that I'm a casual and group sex guy, she feels duped. She has duped herself, but humans are not logical and will prefer to externalize anger. Men are little better. Think of all the blue pill guys who pour attention into a chick, then finally proposition her for sex, then get angry because she "led him on" by letting him pour attention into her. Men learn not to give excess attention to chick we are not having sex with.

I respect Michelle: she knew what she wanted and when she figured out I wasn't going to give it to her, she departed. I liked her, but she was not quite as thin as I would prefer, but she was physically fine. In bed she was average. She was an average girl doing average things. She was probably poorly suited to sex clubs with me. She'd said she'd never been with a woman or had a threesome, which seemed improbable given her background (art school).

She seemed to see a lot of my wholesome-seeming side, like hitting the gym and cooking. She was comically inept in the gym but would go in an attempt to seem like a good life-mate, I think. I've met girls who try to show interest in workouts but who really want to show me how dedicated they are to me, and they never last. With the gym, you have to love the iron discipline for its own sake. If you are trying to use it to get to another goal of some kind, you will very rarely go the distance.

Michelle's younger sister had married very early and just had her first kid, so Michelle appeared to be jealous of her sister and of the attention her sister was getting.

Michelle is also someone I asked to do this a long time ago, before polyamory and open relationships hit mainstream venues. Today, a girl like her will probably have some exposure to ideas around open relationships. I'm writing this on the verge of 2019, and in the last couple years open relationships and alternative sexualities have become far more prominent in the larger media and culture. It seems like girls have some idea about what's available, in a way they didn't have in 2010 or 2013. That could be an incorrect read on my part, but I do feel like the conversation has moved towards non-monogamy, as traditional media gatekeepers have been destroyed by the Internet and people with powerful libidos and sexualities can now speak to the public at large.

Where you live will in part dictate the number of husband hunters you find. In expensive party cities like NYC or LA, you will likely find fewer. In middle America, you will likely find more.

Some girls will say "no" to sex clubs and parties because they don't want to see me f**k another girl. If they say no for that reason, I promise we will only have sex with each other. Often, as they become more comfortable, they'll also relax the "sex with each other only" rule. It reminds me a little of trying to have sex with virgins in high school. Most sexually inexperienced high school girls won't go f**k a guy after one or two dates, unless they're psychologically ready. More commonly, they take weeks or months to f**k, just because they're unused to sexual encounters and sexual expression. They take time to acclimate. Same with non-monogamy. Chicks who are totally unfamiliar will often take time to acclimate. That is why "We only have sex with each other, in this charged atmosphere" is a useful middle ground.

Salesmen often make an "ask" for a prospective client to buy far more than the client will likely buy. Smart salesmen will do this in the hopes of then falling back. "Buy 100 units of this." "No." "Okay, buy ten units." "No." "Okay, how about you try five units, and if you dislike it you can quit, otherwise you'll get another five." "Okay." Same principle here.

I have also dated girls who just say "No." They are not interested. In any circumstances. In the era of *50 Shades of Grey* it is common to depict all chicks as closet nymphomaniacs with intense bondage urges and inner freaks waiting to be let out. In reality not all chicks are like this. Players are more likely to find such chicks, as we're trying to send off "bad boy" and "casual sex" vibes. Chicks who are super vanilla and conventional will want to reject the hard-core player, unless she is up for an adventure at that particular moment.

Seeking Arrangements (SA) girl
* * *

This isn't relevant to most guys's experiences, but years ago I heard about Seeking Arrangements and made an account there, wondering if it would be an eas(ier) way to get laid and what the girls there were like. Early on, I had some crappy SA dates that were oddly similar to crappy regular online dates, except the chicks would also ask for money, but I want to focus on the girl I saw for a long time: she was gorgeous and a very solid 8. Conceivably a low 9, although she didn't dress or act like it. She dressed and acted like a typical college student: jeans, t-shirts, tank-tops, sweatshirts. Okay clothes but she didn't have a lot of experience with or interest in fashion, maybe because she didn't have the money to. Inexperienced but not stupid.

She was a basic girl in many ways but also ready to shed some of her basic habits like TV, boring social networks, and adopt newer, more interesting habits. She didn't behave like the hot girl and at the time I don't think she fully understood how hot she was. Some younger chicks, especially the ones who don't dress with their chests and butts hanging out, don't fully understand their power or how to wield it. Some do, of course, and they can be obnoxious, but this one didn't. I notice that a lot of girls don't figure out how to wield their sexual power until ages 21 – 23.

I'd gone on dates with some other chicks from SA. Some were not as described, the typical online dating problem. One stands out, as she was an outright pro and pretty, but she wanted an outrageous amount of money, and I laughed in her face. She tried to negotiate downwards, but one key to negotiation is to be ready to walk away. I was ready to walk and promptly did. Real pros are usually a little too brittle and distant for my taste. I notably banged two chicks, one multiple times, and gave that one some money, about $200. But when I found SA Girl, I stopped with the SA efforts.

SA Girl looked better than her pictures and was

surprisingly demure. In retrospect, she said she found me deeply intimidating but also someone she could easily talk to. I used a lot of open-ended hopes and dreams and peak experience questions, all of which resonated with her. I think she'd gone out only with guys who wanted to get between her legs as fast as they could. They didn't have good dating or seduction skills, or chose not to use them. Most chicks like to know something of the guy they're going to let inside them, even if they're to be paid. SA Girl really responded to hand-holding, one-minute silent eye contact, closing her eyes and visualizing her dreams and future, those kinds of things. I don't know if I like girls who respond to that kind of thing better, or if girls who like me respond better, but I can get into the "bubble" quickly with it. When it works, it works. We were more compatible than typical people. That sounds like bullshit optimism, but I've been on a lot of gray online dates. Exceptions stand out.

Our first date was a standard drinks date. My message was typical: "Let's get a drink at [bar] and see if we're compatible, and we can go from there." I actively preferred not to attempt a first-night bang, unless she seems game for it, at which point I will calibrate towards the first-night bang. This girl came in a little black dress (very nice, and also unusual) that I later learned she'd borrowed from a friend. I can't say exactly how I knew, but I could sense that she wasn't comfortable in what she was wearing or where she was. It took her time and comfort-building effort on my part to open up. Usually I only do hour-long first dates, but I stayed much longer with her, risking being cast as the provider boyfriend type more than the lover guy. We did a quick kiss before we departed, and I told her we should get together for dinner.

On date two a few days later I picked her up (this was before Uber was common) and made dinner and then we fucked.

She was very nervous and this affected her performance, but I took a very long time with foreplay and warming her up, which allowed her to relax enough to enjoy it. She wanted to stay over and I slipped an envelope with like $200 in it in her purse. She never asked for money. Next time we got drinks together and she was much less inhibited about sex. The connection was still strong.

I may have been able to keep nailing her free, but if a girl is desperate enough for money, she may do both free and paid sex. I said we should do a $500 a month thing and she immediately agreed. That was a lot of money for her and, based on what I've seen since, she doesn't have the personality for sex work (this is a good thing). She got out of the sex-work grind and I got everything I wanted. Again, I could be wrong and for all I know she hooked on the side, but if so she was a master scheduler between school, some normal joe work, and seeing me. It's never a good idea to underestimate the caginess of women, but this one didn't display typical signs of sign of outside action, like sudden absences, unaccounted time blocks, extensive phone guarding, etc. If regular guys underestimate the perfidy and desire of women, some Red Pill guys overestimate them and think all women are routinely, slyly f**king around whenever possible.

As we learned more about each other, SA Girl said she'd only had sex with three guys before, and while I'm skeptical of these kinds of claims, I somewhat believe it... even if you double that number, it's still quite low. She'd dated a guy for two or three years, and she seemed surprised at how long I was willing to go down on her and how attentive I was to her reactions during sex. For example, she had extremely sensitive nipples, and her long-term ex either ignored her boobs or was too rough with her, maybe due to porn. She had bad basic sexual communication skills, which is a sign of inexperience. Some girls can remain in relationships with inept men for very long periods of time and not develop good sexual skills and habits. Others can be trained into good habits by the right guy and become masters of giving and receiving pleasure.

SA Girl had never used sex toys during sex before, and that was a revelation for her. She could come many times by being bent over and having me behind her while she used a vibe on herself. Pretty standard stuff in my world but a total game-changer for her. I think her long-term boyfriend was some combination of young, selfish, and inexperienced. Good sexual communication seemed foreign to her. It took a fair amount of training and openness on my part to get her up to speed, sexually speaking.

Again, to be sure, I can't say the truth about what she was telling me and what I inferred. Why would she stay with a guy who isn't that good in bed for such a long time? Young chicks are often dumb and don't know any better, and she seemed to not know any better. I was much more patient and knowledgeable than other guys she'd been with, and I may have just hit the right girl with the right stuff at the right time. Or she was flattering my ego. But her behaviors seemed to match her words. That level of congruence is not always common. Players know that sometimes a girl is just into you, for whatever reason, and players know to ride that wave when it hits.

To the extent she wanted sexual adventure, she already had it built into our relationship. Even if I had been interested in a monogamous relationship, she would have been too young to attempt one, apart from how we met.

She was willing to go to sex parties with me and was typically the youngest chick there and always in the top three or five in terms of beauty. Like attracts like, as I've written before, and if we found another attractive couple, it was always the couple in the top two or three. As with most things in life, the more value you bring, the more value you get. Some of those couples and women I'm still friends with, long after SA Girl moved away and started some other life (she's married now, or maybe I should say "for now").

In my local scene, I've been seen with multiple extremely hot chicks. That gives me a standing and reputation that has led to many invitations, events, etc. SA Girl in particular made an impression. Lower-level girls can dress themselves up a level or two, but when all the clothes come off we see who a person really is. When the clothes came off, SA Girl was spectacular.

Eventually it was time for SA Girl to move on, and she talked about either staying in my city or me moving with her. The latter was not feasible for me, in terms of work or family. The former was not wise for her: she would come to resent me, and she was too young for a long-term committed relationship. There were a lot of tears on her part, but, just like I say it is wise to catch and release women who want families, it is good to catch and release young girls for whom a long-term relationship is too early. It is better to let a lover go than to wait until the feeling curdles. Many of you will be familiar with people in high school relationships who try to keep it going at separate colleges, or when the guy leaves for college and the girl goes to high school. It almost never works. My typical strategy for this conversation or set of conversations is to explain that she needs to be free, she needs to explore the world, she needs to see what else is in it: if it is meant to be, she will come back and then we will be together.

Spoiler: I am always right and she doesn't come back. Or she comes back for some casual sex but not for a long-term relationship. Even then, when I was seeing SA Girl, I knew that no girl under age 25 or 26 is suitable for a long-term relationship. Guys who think otherwise are typically deluding themselves and setting themselves up for drama and heartbreak. At worse, they marry chicks who are too young and set themselves up for expensive divorce. No thank you!

I don't know what SA is like today, as I've not used it or any other paid site in some time. I assume that, if I stay in the game long term, I will eventually turn towards paid sites again. The Internet is of course filled with 55-year-old guys tagging hot 24-year-old chicks, and, while I know from seeing it that that's possible, it's also hard to do, even for top guys. And that depends on continued health and wealth. A couple months ago, an acquittance died from cancer. He was in his late 30s with two young kids. News like that makes you think about what you want your life to be about.

I can say this particular girl was worth it. We eventually integrated into each other's social networks, which was weird and fun for both of us. She liked being around older and sophisticated people. I liked some of her young hot college friends. The ones who weren't hot and weren't curious about the world I didn't spend any time with, because there was nothing we could offer each other. Some of her friends thought it weird she was dating an older guy and some of them were intrigued.

For guys, SA and related sites are closer to online dating than is commonly realized. It is possible to blow a disgusting amount of money on lame chicks there. It may also be possible to be very cost-effective. I spent far less money on SA Girl than some guys spend on their divorces, their stupid McMansions, and their Teslas… cars are incredibly overrated as far as game and women are concerned. Guys are inept at figuring out what girls truly want and delivering that.

Later, I ran into one of SA Girl's friends on the street and banged her, so that was a nice bit of pre-selection, but the friend was about a high 6 or so. Nothing special apart from the age disparity, but a nice experience whose seeds had been planted years prior. Many players appear to be wanderers, always finding new cities, cold approaching in new places. I've pursued the opposite strategy: living in one place for a long time, knowing it thoroughly, and attempting to build and maintain networks in that place.

The game's end game and the easy win

After the first version of this book had been published, I got an invite to a huge, ticketed private sex party... I've written, "game can be thought of a little bit like chess in that for good players the first 5 – 10 moves are memorized calls and responses and gamed out... the interesting stuff happens midgame." This is an endgame story, making it less valuable than mid-game stories, but I wrote most of it for a private group, so I figured that I'd tell the rest.

At the party, I talked to a gorgeous, short girl who used to be a high-end escort and probably had income that put her in the 99%... not a great conversationalist or was on drugs... some other things about her stood out but are too private to share... asked for kiss when she left, and she said "maybe later." In normal dating asking for the kiss is a bad move, but in this environment it's the way to go. If I had slept with her, she would probably have been in the top five girls I've slept with, ever.

Did an MFM with a couple I know (see the threesome management chapter above): this one happened because I've known them both for years. She is a solid 7, he is probably a male 8... he finds it hard to find the right women, and they are put together well. He's had some of mine before, so it's all good by now you understand reciprocity and balanced equations, and our equations are well-balanced. There is not a "game" story here, or, if there is, it is buried in the years. We are all casual friends who spent some time catching up, then had a theeway. Very intense one, too. Whatever "game" was involved happened long ago.

Much later, I was about to leave and crash, but I saw this girl and had to say hi. I got to chatting and she had great vibes, nice but not astonishing face, and just the best body. 25 or so. We chatted for a while and she noticed my paddle, then asked if I would spank her (I'm the man and I typically lead, so her directness is abnormal but welcome). Of course, baby. We found our way to a more private back area, away from the crowds, and she was just so cute (great, top level super feminine energy) and responsive. Some spanking/paddling, light choking/hair pulling… things moved fast and she was broadcasting horniness… so I just kept going forward, checking in with her at appropriate places… and wow. I didn't think I could rise to the occasion but did it (sometimes verbalizing "I'm not sure I can have sex again" helps me relax into it), and sex with her was just amazing and amazingly fun. Time between "Hi" and f**king was… 20 minutes? 30 minutes? I don't know. It was almost too fast, even for me. I think she'd been marinating in the environment and socializing for a long time and yet hadn't been approached, or properly approached (later I found out that she knew a guy there, a friend of friend, who had been chasing her, but she wasn't into him). Or just right girl right time? I want to give her an 8 due to her body just being packed in all the right ways and feeling fantastic but probably a high 7. Just everything about her felt and seemed right.

I wanted more time to play with her body, but her sex temperature was so high that I felt I couldn't not. We talked about some logistical things related to meeting up again. "feminine energy" isn't discussed as much as it should be. Hers was off the charts. She was like crack. Other girls should take lessons in feminine energy and sounds from her. F**king her was great.

Did not see the former sex worker 9 again.

I wasn't going to include this story in the book because I don't think there's anything new to learn from it... but then I realized that that **is** the lesson: I've been building ecosystem/ connections for many years, and staying in pretty good shape, and it came together in the moment. Maybe I could point out that even s**ts often want to know the guy/guys they're sleeping with... more often than not they do. The first woman came around not because I was a random but because I wasn't. Overall I think I've contributed more value to the community than I've taken, and that was reflected in the private sex party. It was reflected in the invite itself. It was reflected in the people I knew there. It was reflected in the fact that I knew how to be once I was there, and knew where to flirt and where not to. Where to push forward and where to hang back. The interesting things happen in the midgame... but this was the end game, for me, where the value had already been built. The reputation was in place. The beautiful 8 hadn't been approached, or properly approached, and she was ready, so I went for it. I was wandering through the orchard and spotted what might be a ripe fruit... I climbed up... checked it out... turned out to be ripe... and it was good. I had the skills she wanted, and she... well, she had what I wanted. The fruits of the network.

Tried not to drink too much and succeeded... exhausted the next day... I feel a little too old for this shit in some ways to be honest. This FR is late game.... it's about the building of value and discovery and connections over many years. Very few guys can just walk into something like this... you have to know the players involved. The mid-game for this kind of thing is in the rest of the book. Field reports that deal only with the first couple interactions with a woman often aren't interesting because opening moves are pretty well gamed out and most women are going to say "no" to any normal, non-elite guy. Field reports that cover end game, like this one, often aren't interesting because there's not a lot of value building or practice taking place. I've learned to be in the right place at the right time with the right attitudes and that was rewarded. This is a study about reaping wheat, not about growing it (much harder to grow than to reap, or to eat the food made from the wheat). I was surprised by the girl at the end and the speed with which it happened. But the conditions for that had been created over many years. I've had this happen before, but this girl was just f**kin hot, and she's relatively to new to the scene/community. In some ways I got lucky, but you know how the harder you work, the luckier you seem to get?

The psychology of unlocking abundance

An anonymous player I know read this book and has implemented many of its ideas and strategies. He says,

Group sex has fundamentally shifted my thoughts about Red Pill and seduction. I cannot understate the change in me. It really does feel like a shift from scarcity to abundance.

I know this feeling and yet no other writing players I'm aware of are tapping non-monogamy and groups. Threesome and group sex fantasies are very common among both men and women, as women themselves attest, but most women are passive and lack the leadership necessary to make their fantasies reality. Very few women know guys who can pull off executing these fantasies, so, if you become that guy, you are by definition not a commodity guy. Women are bombarded by commodity guys with basic or no sex skills, and a guy who can unlock their dirtier fantasies is not that guy. If you tap into the sex club world, you will also end up unlocking a pool of girls who are pre-selected for liking to f**k a lot... and then you can f**k them.

Women have the fantasy, but the group-sex reality usually needs deep coordination between the participants, especially for MFM. The threesome management guide probably understates the degree to which coordination is important. Ideally all the players should cooperate and coordinate, but the temptation to defect remains potent in many threesome situations, and it often happens that one party is less active during some parts than the other two parties. This can lead to feelings of isolation and being left out, particularly because most threesomes happen between an established couple and a third person. The third person often brings new relationship energy (NRE) in with them.

After an MFM or FMF, the aftercare for the girl is super important. Many girls will experience sub-drop, and the girl may be susceptible to feelings of worthlessness, low sexual marketplace value, disgust, regret, etc. The girl may need reaffirmation that she is a good person, that sexuality is fun and normal, that she is not dirty or degraded, and that she's not just a f**k-toy for men. That means she probably needs to be held, cuddled, chatted with, etc. The man should check in with her the next day, in person if possible. It's a good idea to do a non-sexual or low-sexual date as soon as possible, like getting coffee or going for a walk. This allows her to process the intensity of the group sex situation and feel that her normal life is not disturbed by what she may feel are depraved fantasies.

All of these challenges can be overcome and mitigated, but the novice group-sex initiate often doesn't anticipate them. I don't think I anticipated them effectively. I also didn't anticipate how it was possible to <u>combine non-monogamy, game, and sex clubs to unlock abundance and commodification</u>.

Another player says,

I thought you need to be an experienced player to do threesomes and group sex and now I organised MFM is less than four months in a game with a first regular after four months dry spell. Wtf is going on?

I can understand it... and that is part of the reason I like it... and also part of the reason I think the rest of my game has improved... I genuinely don't give a fuck if any individual girl is into me or not, which makes them more into me, and protects my vibe/state during cold streaks. I know that I'll end up getting laid one way or another... so if she wants these peak experiences, she needs to enter my world. That's kind of the attitude, or the frame. Many women reject the gift... and that's fine... most people's lives are kind of crappy.

I want to emphasize that I care a lot about the women in my life who I choose and who choose me, and with whom I have a tight bond. Many guys get hurt or angry when a strange women rejects them. That's the wrong way to think about it, although I understand how desperation and horniness drives guys to think that way. The woman who offers a swift rejection gives you the gift of your time and <u>attention</u>, to better deploy them. Time is always finite, and one modern tragedy is the way people waste it on social media.

The player who organised the MFM also substituted (some) knowledge for experience. **That is the beauty and magic of books... they accelerate learning**. Reading a book is no perfect substitute for experience, as should be obvious, but the player who's read it has the intellectual and social framework for implementing group sex and non-monogamy ideas. I had to build up those things from scratch.

I think most guys think threesomes "just happen" after a bunch of drinking and lucky circumstances. You are taking "just happens" and making an industrial process or algorithm out of it. Once you have the fundamental, you know what to do. Discovering the algorithm is hard, but implementing it is (relatively) easy. This book allows guys to get past the innovation phase and towards the engineering/ implementation phase.

One theme you've seen running through this book is about markets, supply, and demand. Magnum tweeted out, The Dating Market: Thesis Overview, about dating market dynamics... "A conservative estimate of the percentage of new relationships begun online in 2019 is at least 65%, but likely over 75%." "The social costs of rejecting a potential mate are now likewise effectively zero, making introductions within existing social groups (friends, family friends, church, etc.) structurally inferior propositions given significant social and reputational risk in the event of an adverse outcome."

The age dynamic creates significant inter-age cohort competition in the female population and increased overall competition in the male population. This can be conceptualized as the market becoming more efficient, which naturally leads to many market participants anecdotally expressing unhappiness with the status quo as they incorrectly identify an inability to produce low effort excess returns as the circumstances being "unfair." Basically, the same thing is happening in the dating market as is happening in the Hedge Fund market: things are getting more efficient, very few are pleased about it, and there are lots of strange advice books, blogs, and videos coming out.

* * *

For top guys, women become a commodity... something this author has missed.

<u>We could say</u>, "Sometimes it seems to me that a good unified theory of modern society's anxieties might be 'everything is too efficient and it's exhausting.'" Dating is more efficient in some ways, but less efficient in others. Most chicks can't accurately assess a guy through his online bullshit. Most guys however can accurately assess about how hot a chick is. So chicks have lots of choices without good ways of navigating those choices. This seems like a detour, but the market for basic guys is flooded.

The market for guys who can make a woman's sexual fantasies come true remains thin. Most guys can't do this. I'm teaching guys how not to be like most guys. I don't know, maybe in 10 years all guys will have threesomes and group sex in their quivers, and it won't be a significant differentiator. For right now, today, it sure is. I am helping guys get out of the efficient markets and into inefficient markets for making fantasies happen. If every guy is on Tinder he will be judged accurately and harshly as a commodity, but if he is doing daygame, building his value, and offering enticing non-commodity experiences, well then he's going to offer unusual value.

I also think most guys and chicks are doing online dating poorly, but that is a rant for another time.

New thread, a player had an MFM and then worked through the aftermath of it,

We did a debrief today and discussed the good, the bad and the ugly of the MFM. One lesson learnt for me was having a second crack at [girl] while [player 1] was in the shower. We cleared that up and agreed no more sex unless he or I are back in the room with our main girl.

Personally I'm not worried about sex happening with the main girl while I'm not in the room, provided that I trust the other guy. But I understand where these rules come from. In addition, applying this kind of business logic or practice to sex is also how to build skills rapidly. Most guys, especially younger guys who have not been in the work world, are not familiar with these kinds of practices. There are different formal methodologies for this, like six sigma, but they are pretty similar. Smart businesses know they are key to rapidly building skills and improving product, service, etc. There is no reason they cannot or should not also be applied to seduction... or in this case to group sex. Most of us have ego defenses that inhibit us from getting honest negative feedback, but the good/bad/ugly mechanism or mechanisms like it help us overcome ego defenses and work to maximize skill improvement.

After intense group sex experiences it's often good to run through these kinds of things to determine what limits and boundaries are there as well as how to make them better next time. Each individual and couple needs to work out their own rules and principles, and I can't do that for them.

Overall, these players are hitting many of the expected milestones, so it's positive to see that my experience doesn't seem to be unique but instead is part of a pattern that is replicable by others.

Over time, the sex club and party worlds can become a big part of a guy or couple's social world. The friends I made there carry over into every day life, doing every day things like going to movies, or museums, or hikes. Normal people aren't sex machines: sex is a big part of their life, but not the only part, and to know someone properly, you have to know them outside of party world. At the same time, some of my regular friends, who I meet from work or other events, often learn about my sex party proclivities, and if they're sufficiently interested, I'll tell them they can come. Social worlds can wind up merging this way.

I don't announce to everyone that I go to sex parties, but I don't hide it, either. It's part of who I am, like playing basketball or writing poetry might be part of who someone else. A guy who writes poetry may mention he does, and see if someone else wants to talk about how great Seamus Heaney is. All conversations are in part about one person extending a topic and seeing if the other person responds. Socially weird people don't read other people's signs and often end up isolated. Two people who don't get along with each other may have very different interests.

Sex is so encompassing an activity that people who do it with each other get closer, fast, as I've mentioned. Letting another guy enter your woman is an extremely intimate act, as is you entering his. This kind of intimacy can bond people together, leading to general social closeness. The power of these bonds mean they can wind up weakening other bonds. I'm not saying this is good, but I am saying it's something I've noticed.

The cadence of sex clubs, parties, and non-monogamous dating can vary. Some people will occasionally drop by a sex party every few months, with their long-term partner, for a bit of variety. A few will want to go on dates every week, or twice a week, although that's usually exhausting. I've been in periods that can last for months when these activities engulf my life. I've also been in periods when I'm dating a woman and either not dating anyone else or minimally dating anyone else. I write this present update in November 2021, and for the last two years I've done minimal dating of other women and couples, because I'm at that point in life when doors are shutting (often quietly), opportunities are going away, and the paths I choose are the ones I'll have to walk. A twenty-year old has an incredibly wide angle of potential paths and changes in front of him. People say "age is just a number," and there's truth to that, but it's also a lie: the older a person gets, the less he can make radical changes and expect them to take. His formerly single friends have kids, get married (sometimes in that order), rearrange their lives. The way women and potential friends respond to him changes. He builds skill, or doesn't, and reaps the rewards from building unique skills—or doesn't. If it takes ten years to truly master a field, a man only has a handful of potential skills he can master in his life, and most don't even master one.

Sex clubs and parties can be all-encompassing, which has positive elements and negative. They can unlock true abundance. They also, like all things, entail trade-offs, and I've tended to live for medium-term relationships of a few months to a year, which is a statement about my own psychology and proclivities, not a recommendation to others. I've done some extreme things, but it's hard to generalize about what it's been like to be me during this period of my life. I've had periods when I've been sleeping with three women in a week, for many weeks in a row. I've had periods when I've been focusing on my career. I've learned a lot, and now I'm trying to pass that knowledge to others.

CHAPTER THREE

Conclusion

Most works about open relationships versus this one

Most texts about open relationships are written by people, often women, with no knowledge of evolutionary biology and no understanding about why and how jealousy evolved. Books like *The Ethical Slut*, *More Than Two*, and *Sex At Dawn* have their uses, especially when you want to convert a girl and need a book to hand her. She can read it and probably won't see the book's flaws. Those books also want to ignore the operant realities in the mating and dating markets, and they are politically correct. They ignore or discount important ideas about differing individual sexual market values among men, among women, and between men and women. Put crudely, most men want "younger, hotter, tighter." Most women want men who are tall and fit, yes, but also prestigious, dominant, or some combination of prestigious and dominant. Humans are unusual in that we have many differing status hierarchies, and a guy who doesn't like his place in one status hierarchy will often try a different one; it is not an error that many actors and musicians are short: they are more motivated to try to succeed than their taller competitors.

This book is an attempt to correct the non-monogamy books that are wrong and missing male perspective as well as evolutionary biology. Because few books are written from a man's perspective today, this book will offend a lot of women who don't know anything true about the male experience. This book is also designed educate guys with game, but it's also an attempt to rescue open relationships from the consistent, blue pill, female-first framing one sees in the larger media. Women remain the gatekeepers of sex, while men remain the gatekeepers of commitment. A sex party that gets hot women attending regularly will be amazing. A sex party that cannot attract and protect hot women will not last. Running parties demands incredible social skills, logistical skills, and tact. But the rewards of running a party are clear, in that other people bring sexy girls to you to get f**ked. The scene turns on hot women.

Women know, instinctively, that guys are less likely to commit to sexually adventurous women, because those women are more likely to leave the man, cuckold him, and bear another man's child. But women have their own set of sexual drives and desires, many of which call for novelty, bisexuality, attention, and group sex. I've mentioned Nancy Friday's book *My Secret Garden* earlier; it's an early elaboration of these desires. Game-aware men can harness and activate those desires. This book focuses on a subset of open relationships, related to group sex and sex parties. There are other kinds, though I don't think they're well-suited to players. It's also possible for players to agree to be in a "polyamorous" relationship with a woman, with the understanding that she's just a friends-with-benefits or occasional lover, while the guy keeps up the game with new women.

It could be said that I've been "researching" this book for

ten years, although I didn't consciously think about my experiences as research, and I didn't begin to articulate what I've learned until recently. Then, as I began to explain what I've done, and I began to see many misconceptions in reaction to what I've done, I started to realize that I've learned a lot of subtle lessons that outsiders or those with minimal experience don't understand and often can't understand.

Those outsiders include the semi-journalists who work for content mills. Today, popular content mills include Bustle, Elite Daily, Vice, New York Magazine, Allure, and, I'm sure, others. Tomorrow, some of those sites will have died and others will have taken their place. A typical media article from these kinds of outlets is like, "I went to a sex party and here's what happened, LOL," written by some chick whose goal is to evince a superior attitude. She does a quick online search, she finds some of the articles by other inexperienced girls like her, she finds a club, she goes to it with her boyfriend, she writes the article the next day, she moves on to the next article she's getting paid $50 to write. I've been in the scene for a decade, sometimes more deeply involved and sometimes less, and I now understand a lot that was hidden to me when I got started. Those 1,000-word popular content articles have some utility in that they encourage women to be sex positive and try attending sex parties, but they miss a lot too. I'm filling in the gaps and explaining to players who this can work for them.

Monogamy is also failing due to the prevalence of Facebook, iPhones, and other technologies that make it far too easy to surreptitiously hook up with exes. When a woman has been with a man for a couple years and is going through a tough or boring period with him, she can easily start a Facebook chat with her old boyfriends or crushes. The very low friction required for women to begin an affair today is corrosive to conventional relationships. For most women, social media is like crack, and most women lack the willpower to say "no." This world of easy sex-on-demand is revealing all the cracks in the facade of monogamy. Social media is revealing the many problems with elite institutions, a topic dealt with in *The Revolt of the Public* by Martin Gurri—a book players should read, though it is not directly applicable to the game.

Social media weakens existing relationships, increases non-monogamy, and also makes it easier to discover cheating. In this environment, consensual non-monogamy makes more sense than ever. Many guys fantasize about a monogamous relationship with a woman, but they fail to realize that few women will remain in a long-term monogamous relationship with them. We're only just now coming to terms with the way social media tears apart relationships of all kinds. But as old relationships and bonds dissolve, new ones will take their place. What will those look like? What should those look like?

As we learn about why and how monogamy doesn't work, we also have to ask what comes after monogamy. This book is a partial answer to that question, although I haven't framed it as such until now.

One takeaway for players who don't want a committed relationship is simple: it's possible to use sex clubs to extend relationships that would otherwise fizzle out at the point when the girl is looking for something more serious. A girl who truly wants marriage and family will reject the player, but many girls don't know what they want, or oscillate between wanting a family guy and a hot player guy. A sufficiently hot player guy may retain the girl for months or years even if she thinks, when she is not sexually aroused, that she wants a family.

This book contains many generalizations, and you will find exceptions to those generalizations. Patterns remain over time. Statistical patterns remain in the face of outliers. In the game, you'll also find exceptions but more often you'll also find patterns. Most couples are composed of a man and woman who are somewhat close to the same "level" at their respective sexual hierarchies. They are image-matched. Relationships that don't have some amount of evenness (you could even call it "reciprocity") tend to fall apart. In non-monogamy, it's possible to cadge some value, but that's unusual. If you want to have a better time in the non-monogamous world, you need to up your value and improve your value-delivery mechanism, just like the game more generally. That's why I say that non-monogamy is just a special case of the game.

In addition, this book doesn't present short cuts or attempt to make non-monogamy sound like "the easy way" to lots of fun sex with a variety of partners. Finding a good partner, attending events, screening other couples or women, following up, and going on dates can be a lot of work. Despite the work, I would argue that, once the system is set up and the principles understood, it can run pretty smoothly. There are no shortcuts.

Sometimes, things will be smooth… you meet a woman or couple you like, get their number, and they respond, "Yes, let's meet for a date on Thursday at the bar you've suggested." You go on a date, come back, and have sex. In this book, I'm trying to cover a lot of edge-case scenarios for the sake of thoroughness. The downside of thoroughness is that the scenario can sound more challenging than it may turn out to be in real life.

What might seem overwhelming at first becomes second nature, commonplace, over time: it's like riding a motorcycle… the first time you're on it you're like, "Jesus Christ, how am I gonna constantly shift, and throttle, and brake, and throttle again, and turn, all at the same time…"

But soon enough you stop thinking about it, it becomes automatic.

Like learning anything, it takes some time to process and internalize what's happening... understanding what I've described in this book took me a couple years and a couple relationships to properly see. The book is a map, so guys who have read it will spend less time wandering in the wilderness and will be familiar with some landmarks, but the map is not the territory, and exploring a new place will include some confusion.

This book won't appeal to every man, and it is an open work: it is up to you, the reader, to complete it, by implementing the ideas within. Mastering the game, rather than relying on random chance and half-cocked assumptions, does not appeal to most men. Of those men who become good at seduction, only a minority will pursue the open-relationship path. It has proven a rich and fruitful path to me, and it has provided a solution to the, "Where is this going?" talk that ends most uncommitted relationships. For the overwhelming majority of men, relationships entail trade-offs. Exceptionally attractive, famous men may be able to relatively easily have as many one-night stands and short relationships with attractive women as they want. For the rest of us, there is only the struggle, the game, the practice, the defeats, and, too rarely, the victories.

If you enjoyed *Sex Clubs, Non-Monogamy, and Game*, then you should read my novel, *The Good Girl*, which is available at the link and at Amazon. Anyone who's read this whole book will enjoy *The Good Girl*:

> He meets Maggie on the street, cold reading her like she's a tarot card and hoping she's entertained enough not just to say she'll go on a date, but to

actually appear on it.

She's between boyfriends and more open to men than usual, but wary enough of a random man's birdsong, however compelling the initial birdsong might appear.

He's got a secret plan, she's got justified suspicions, and the game that unfolds is, in some sense, The Game—the universal game all men and women play.

The tension between them can't be resolved without destroying the game, and yet the tension and uncertainty draws them both together, propelling them towards unpredictable ends that will leave both changed, forever.

You'll see some of the ideas here, developed further there.

Acknowledgements

This book is dedicated to my ideal reader and frequent interlocutor Nash, https://daysofgame.com.

Thank you to all the guys who have read it and provided feedback: Magnum, Jake, Craig, Yohami, and whoever I might have forgotten.

Thank you to every girl I have ever f**ked. And to every girl who turned me down: I learned something from you, too.

Thank you to every writer who has ever meant something to me. This book continues the conversation. Today, many of the most interesting writers don't write or publish under their own names.

Onward.